Vinnie Woods has embarked on a fledgling writing journey by writing this book, *My Black Dog Keeps Biting,* which was promised because of his lifetime struggle living with a devastating illness—depression. His discovery of a real passion for writing, quite accidently it would be fair to say, came at a time when he had to finally stand up and face his demons head on. His love of the written word has definitely gripped his senses as he has now fallen into the world of children's books as well.

This book is dedicated to Sian – my wife, my whole world, my best friend and soul mate. She's the real reason I've been able to write and finish this written account of my life. Without her constant love and support, this publication would never have seen the light of day.

Vinnie Woods

My Black Dog
Keeps Biting

AUSTIN MACAULEY PUBLISHERS™

LONDON • CAMBRIDGE • NEW YORK • SHARJAH

A CIP catalogue record for this title is available from the British Library.

ISBN 9781528987387 (Paperback)
ISBN 9781528987394 (ePub e-book)

www.austinmacauley.com

First Published (2021)
Austin Macauley Publishers Ltd
25 Canada Square
Canary Wharf
London
E14 5LQ

To Margaret – thank you for all your help and support that you've so kindly given to me over the very many years that our paths have met. I will always be indebted to you.

To Isobel – you were there to listen and empathise. You helped me beat my demons. I can never thank you enough.

To Mel – your words got me started, all I can say is thank you.

Foreword

I feel privileged to have been asked to write this foreword to Philip's book.

I have travelled with him for much of his journey, witnessing his endeavours to overcome the effects of the trauma in his childhood, the years of constant fight and struggle with depression, the impact on his relationships, several attempts to end his life as he searched for meaning and freedom from "blame."

I believe he has now found that freedom. He has written about his journey in a way that will give hope and encouragement to others still struggling with their demons.

I truly respect and admire this young man and his brave and courageous determination and I commend his book to anyone on a similar journey.

That it helps Sian, his family and friends and others will be the accolade for him.

– Margaret Corkeran RMN.CPN

Chapter One
The Straw and the Camel!
October 2017

Fuck! What's happening? I've been here before I thought, but this was an unfamiliar experience, far more intense and debilitating than any previous scary episode. I could feel myself shutting down which was definitely a normal reaction to one of my many falls but this was different, very different.

I couldn't assemble rationality for love nor money and physically I felt fragile and weak from my addled head to the tips of my toes. Every living cell in my body was screaming abuse at me. This was no ordinary episode of depression. What the hell was happening, was this the end, was it finally going to kill me? The irony was not lost having survived seven suicide attempts.

I find myself lying in bed attempting to shut out the world but deep in the knowledge that something was very wrong with me. I try to decipher my jumbled thoughts and analyse why this is so different. Have all these years of constant fight and struggle finally taken their toll, is this it? It certainly feels that way.

The gut-churning and stomach-wrenching feeling like an army of malignant beasts pulling at my insides and they won't be satisfied until they've completely disembowelled me. Nausea has stepped up to the highest level which is impossible to describe and the usual descending black cloud is magnified to a full-blown storm. I try to focus on the pattern of the ceiling to stop my head spinning around like a tornado and lifting my head off the pillow is nigh on impossible. This is not good! Weakness is a common symptom for me when I get ill which is difficult to accept as I pride myself on being a strong geezer. Now, I feel my strength is akin to a baby. Fucking hell!

I have no recollection of how many hours passed but a wave of deepening realisation that yep, this is the end of the line washed over me as my mind and body finally gave up. It was tired of decades of the constant daily fight and was telling me that enough was enough, no more.

I knew that this time I was fucked, done, totally spent with nothing left to give or take. As usual, I refuse to communicate with anybody but this time I knew I had to deal with this deadly imposter once and for all. I had to do it for my health, my sanity and for my long-suffering family. In particular, my absolute rock and soulmate, Sian, my wife.

The Poem

The poem and its words came to me during one of my many dark episodes and to this day I have absolutely no idea where it came from. I had never attempted to write a poem before and believed I hadn't a poetic or creative bone in my body.

It was approximately three years ago, even before the thought of writing this book that the words came to me and were indelibly marked on my brain from then onwards. Who sent them or why they came to me were puzzling for some time. But I have come to the conclusion that higher forces were at work and they were responsible for unearthing these few but vitally important words.

I say important because the black dog gave me the title for my book and ultimately provided the courage and initial platform to begin putting pen to paper about my life and consequent experiences.

My Black Dog Keeps Biting My Black Dog

You might know me well, but not as much as you think
Because I always have this black dog by my side every day,
who just won't go away.
We will walk through fields, over hills and into towns and
cities, but when I can no longer walk anymore, we find
ourselves back at my front door.
I tell him that it's time for him to go and I hope and pray that
this becomes so.
When I awake the next day, I hear the sound of barking, I go
downstairs to see, who it is that's beckoning me.
Who should be there?
It's my faithful black dog, fixing me with his stare.

Chapter Two

What! Me, Write a Book?
March 2018

Sian had asked a work colleague and friend, Mel, to pay me a visit as she was qualified in massage therapy, which I had always found helpful in the past for managing my depression. It felt a little strange as I had not met her before, but I found Mel to be very friendly and incredibly easy to talk to. It also turns out that she's a bit witchy and spiritual. She won't mind me saying that!

During the massage, the conversation evolves and the subject of my depression arises. I found myself talking openly and in-depth about my illness and my life in minute detail to this person whom I had not met before. Mel listened intently and suddenly interjected with "you should write a book on this subject, Phil, you have first-hand experience and years of extensive knowledge. It would be cathartic and who knows who else you may help."

It was like a light bulb moment, Mel was right. Perhaps I could put down on paper my immeasurable experiences and deeply ingrained thoughts. In the past, others had suggested I do the same but until now I had thought it a ridiculous idea and had never taken the idea seriously. Maybe at that time, I lacked the confidence and belief that I had the ability to knuckle down and write an historic account of my life which I knew would unearth previously buried sad and painful events.

For whatever bizarre reason, Witching Mel had given me the conviction that in fact, I could do this which immediately boosted my morale and confidence. I don't make this statement lightly as it will come as a huge surprise, dare I say shock, to those who know me that I am a budding author of a book they may well decide to read. In addition, to think I could seriously help other people suffering mental health issues feels extraordinarily empowering but equally frightening as that isn't without great responsibility.

I guess what I want to get across is that depression does not discriminate and can affect anybody at any time from whichever walk of life you may be from. I'm just your average man in the street and if I can help by sharing my experiences, then writing this book will be worth every effort. Opening my soul and exposing my flaws and weaknesses feels somewhat daunting and terrifying but if I can help just one individual manage this fucking horrible illness once and for all, then my work will have been done.

I also think that for those who know me well may think I have finally lost it and taken leave of my senses. Let's hope not.

Chapter Three

Broken, Phil Has Finally Left the Building

The fallout from the cataclysmic event of October 2017 had left me with massive scars, both mentally and physically. Such was the sheer power of my depressive episode that even as I write these words, I am completely unable to recall the exact day of my meltdown. I am only aware that it was October, such is my blurred, frazzled memory of the time.

I do remember, however, exactly how I felt in the days and early weeks following my sudden descent into the dark, black pit of despair. I have had many experiences over the years of being completely and utterly zombiefied (is that even a word!) but this time was totally different. It was on a level that I can only imagine must have been like for those poor desperate souls who were subjected to a surgical lobotomy years ago. I was out of it, fucked, a barely walking empty shell of my former self.

I vaguely recall shutting the world out and talking to my bed for two maybe three days, which was my usual routine whenever this bastard illness struck. All I do know is that much of this time was spent asleep. Feeling tired has always been one side effect of an episode but it never ceases to amaze me how much I'm able to sleep but still feel completely washed out. Again, I refuse to talk to Sian or anybody for that matter. I completely shut down and refuse any attempt of interaction because I feel so weak and cannot find the energy to even speak.

When I did awaken, I'd find myself staring at the ceiling, ruminating negative and destructive thoughts, the kind that drives you crazy and have no purpose or positive outcome. Eventually, I drag my sorry arse out of bed probably because I'm sick of sleeping and staring at the bloody Artex ceiling. Besides, I was dying for a cup of rosy which is a bit of a yardstick for me as it normally indicates that I'm feeling slightly better.

Walking down the stairs was an incredible effort, my legs were like jelly and I still felt nauseous and spaced out. As crazy as it sounds, even making the tea was proving somewhat of a challenge. I turned on the TV to catch up on the sports news and although I was watching, nothing was registering or made sense.

I had to remind myself that I was just coming out of the mother of all episodes and it dawned on me that I hadn't had my medication for two, three maybe even four days.

So, I'm sitting staring at the football news and my swede is absorbing absolutely nothing. Football is a massive part of my life as Sian will testify to but I may as well have been watching a blank screen for all the good it was doing. This carried on into the following week. I couldn't concentrate on the simplest of tasks and this began to manifest in frustration and anger, especially towards Sian, which was totally unfair and bang out of order but I couldn't snap out of it.

I wasn't coping at all and must have been a right royal pain in the arse to live with. Obviously, the little dialogue I had with Sian was not the best but this evil bastard illness was winning at the time and try as I might, I was losing the battle.

I am more than happy to repeat myself here to reiterate that Sian has always been my rock and soulmate and did not deserve to be treated in the manner she did and for now I want to say I'm sorry Sian and I love you.

Chapter Four

Still Broken, Crawling My Way Back

An obvious statement of fact I know but it has to be said that I was only able to take one day at a time in the days and weeks that followed my meltdown. After two or three weeks, my mood did start to improve albeit very slowly. Everyday tasks became easier although I did struggle with concentration particularly when I read. So, I started to listen to music again as in addition to finding it uplifting, music is one of my passions. My loss of appetite is another symptom I suffer with when I am struck down by this horrible illness. Immediately after an episode, I will eat next to nothing for several days and slowly introduce two meals a day as my appetite begins to return slowly.

Time passes and Sian and I are talking more but the situation is causing an undercurrent of strain, thankfully not in a hostile way. During settled periods in our relationship, Sian and I are loving, happy and rarely argue but presently, the tension is palpable and neither of us like it one bit. The depressive event has knocked us both for six and were struggling to deal with the fallout, both emotionally and physically. It has left us drained and struggling to visualise our future.

Although I'm starting to feel better as the days pass, I know that I'm far from 100% fit whereas normally, I would shake the fall off within a week or so. This time it seems I am moving nowhere quickly. My confidence feels shot and nagging thoughts still surface in my brain. However hard I try to think positive and dismiss these thoughts, the fucking demons are still winning the battle and it will be a further six months before I start winning the war.

When you have suffered from depression for most of your life, it is very hard to employ a tool inside your head that can alter your train of thought. Deep, ingrained thinking makes this difficult to address and takes considerable effort and time before you notice any encouraging changes. Whilst I have been fortunate enough to have many positive aspects of my life, I can categorically say to you that most of my memories tend to be negative and upsetting.

Days go by and before I know where I am, it's November and my 52nd birthday. Not that I had much enthusiasm for that day, to be honest! I remember thinking am I still going to be here another year from now? Will I still be fighting and sending myself mad with sheer frustration? Will I be any nearer to beating the demons that I have been plagued with for so long? When will it ever fucking end?

I don't know if I have the strength to do this for another year!

As yet I have not mentioned my work, but it goes without saying that it has been impossible to carry out my job as a taxi driver/chauffeur. It requires complete concentration to remember routes, drive safely and strangely be able to function as a counsellor for many passengers who use you as a verbal punch bag to spill their tales of woe. I am a million miles away from being strong enough to cope with this psychologically now or in the near future.

The next couple of weeks follow the same vein, but at least now I have been able to kick start my gym work again. Up until this point, I have felt too weak to contemplate training even though I have really missed my sessions, there was absolutely no way I was up to it and probably would have injured myself in the process. I have weight trained regularly for over thirty years, not as a serious bodybuilder, just to keep myself fit really. Due to a serious football injury, I had to give up playing and investing in gym equipment set up in the garage provided an alternative means of maintaining my fitness. I cannot overstress the benefits of exercise and I can testify that it has helped me greatly over the years in battling depression. It kept me going when perhaps I might have fallen by the wayside much sooner than I actually did.

Another small step to my recovery was being able to face the world again. Popping to the local shop had been the extent of my travels as I just wasn't up to going out socially. Sian and I slowly began to have a few beers with close friends again, something I really enjoy doing and mixing with others always made me happy. On one such occasion with very good friends of ours, it seemed an opportune moment to talk to them about my meltdown and I wanted to explain to them the sheer hurricane force that had ripped through me. They are both more than aware with my battle of depression as they have been witnessing it, rearing its ugly head on several occasions.

I think many people find understanding depression difficult and sometimes when you are seen to be enjoying yourself, it is difficult to appreciate the turmoil a person is enduring.

I love the bones of this couple and they appeared pleased when I had explained the seriousness of my situation and I am eternally grateful to them both for confirming their support for me. If there is one thing I have learnt, it is that you need to talk to your loved ones and keep them in the loop. They deserve to know and the flipside to this is that you are more likely to continue receiving the support you need. Communication is key!

Thank you so much, Lec and Lisa!

Chapter Five

Beginning to Find My Legs

I'm functioning a little better, but I am acutely aware that this imposter has not left me.

Just what the fuck is it? Why haven't you left me yet? Is this permanent and as good as it gets from now on? I fucking hope not as I am not strong enough to beat this if it carries on for much longer, that is for sure.

I'm becoming concerned as this underlying feeling has not got any worse but has not improved either. Usually, when I feel a decline, I have always been fortunate to have the immediate support of my mental health nurse, Margaret, but unfortunately, she has sadly been poorly and been on long-term sickness from work. A privilege many people with mental health issues do not have due to lack of finance and resources. I called my GP practice to enquire if Margaret had returned to work which she hadn't and was offered an appointment with a GP whom I had seen several times previously. He's a lovely guy and had always treated me with understanding and respect, which has not always been the case! I explained my situation to the receptionist and Dr O called me in no time at all. After a lengthy conversation, we decided between us to change one of my medications. I stopped taking pregabalin and commenced on mirtazapine to have alongside my usual duloxetine. Dr O asked me to see how I got on over the next few weeks and to get back to him should I experience any problems. He also advised me that Margaret would be returning to work in the near future which lifted my spirits as I was beginning to lose hope of getting the help I so desperately needed.

I was able to carry on training, but my energy levels were not as they normally would be and I felt as if I was just going through the motions. Sian reassured me by affirming that some exercise was still better than no exercise at all and we began to seek out areas where we could go for regular walks. Something we had always enjoyed. I can strongly recommend exercise to help combat depression as it can really clear your head and improve your mood so go and enjoy. As a nurse, Sian has explained that there is a scientific reason, but I'm not even going to try to reiterate it!

I was beginning to feel guilty about placing the financial pressure onto Sian's shoulders and although I have always had a strong work ethic, this illness has forced me to take time out which had definitely increased over the years. It caused me concern that Sian may harbour resentment towards me as she took the full strain financially and psychologically. I was used to having money and contributing as I could towards our living costs but I was now unable to do this, leaving me feeling like a complete sponger. As usual, I needn't have worried as when I told Sian exactly how I felt she was brilliant and reinforced her commitment to me getting well and beating this illness. Crucially, she also told me not to put pressure on myself to get better.

That fucking demon was still feeding those negative and damaging thoughts.

You're a fucking leech, a sponger. When are you gonna get your act together? It's not what she really thinks!

The logical side of your brain tells you that the above thoughts are totally false, but that bastard demon never gives up, poking and prodding your brain with a bloody jackhammer. I just wish you would fuck off.

Sian and I began to go out more from time to time which helped break up the monotony of being home. I have tried to keep my mind occupied by weight training, listening to music and reading. Lots and lots of reading! I haven't minded being at home so much, to be honest as I have been content in taking every day as it comes and not overdoing it just in case of the dreaded relapse. In the past, I would have gone stir crazy. Again, throughout this period, Sian continued with her fabulous ongoing support and is an absolute godsend.

Here we go again, my demon must be bored.

Why is she with me when I bring so much shit to her door? She would be better off without me.

I don't want to bring her any more hurt. I gate-crashed her life more than sixteen years ago with this horrible illness and she doesn't deserve this. It makes me feel ashamed. Again, I'm sorry, Sian.

Chapter Six

Kicking the Leaves

It's autumn, the beginning of November and the crisp leaves are falling from the trees and hitting the cold ground. I remember as a small child, running and kicking huge piles of dead leaves and even jumping in headfirst. I remember how much fun this was and not having a care in the world. How amazing would that be to feel this way as an adult? I think just everyone would love to go back and be a child again even if for just one day. The start of November brought about my 52nd birthday not that it was bringing me any joy whatsoever. I really didn't want to celebrate the fact that yet another had slipped me by in the blink of an eye.

All my attention was on getting well again and I didn't have the energy or enthusiasm for any dramas or distractions. I continued to take one day at a time, which in reality felt like Groundhog Day. Thinking back, although Sian and I were getting on much better, we were basically treading water. We continued to keep motivated by going out for our walks and the occasional night out with friends, but I felt fragile and liable to break at any moment. I carried on exercising even though my heart often wasn't in it and the mental and physical tiredness was becoming the norm for me. I had the urge to train harder and at a level, I felt I was still able to achieve but the exhaustion sapped my muscles. Weight plates occasionally found themselves thrown in sheer frustration. Sorry neighbours! But try as hard as I could, I was just going through the motions and becoming increasingly frustrated with the whole situation.

This is pissing me right off now!
When will this tiredness ever end?
Am I going to feel like an old man forever?

The days seem to drift by tediously. I'm functioning but probably only at 50% of my normal, well self. Whatever that is? I honestly can't remember what 'normal' really feels like. My fuzzy head resembles the times I've attempted to stop taking the medication which left me floating in a parallel universe. Fortunately, I got wind of my mental health nurse, Margaret, returning to work so I called her in November to explain my current state of mind and how I was really struggling again. We arranged an urgent appointment which I had to wait a couple of weeks for but I was just so relieved to be able to see her again. Margaret had been on long-term sick leave and not having her support had been extremely difficult.

In the middle of November, we paid a visit to our great friend, Dr Andrew Davies to meet his new partner, Kate. We made the pleasurable journey with our other good friends, Lee and Lisa in their brand new 'Beamer'. We met the lovely Dr Davies shortly after moving into our first rented home and he was our neighbour. Andy has since retold the horrific impressions we gave to his then partner. Sian and I became known as the 'tattooed thug and bleach blonde bimbo'. How rude! How funny! We may be at different ends of the intellectual spectrum, but essentially, we found ourselves getting on incredibly well and had a mutual interest in enjoying ourselves to the full. The summer of 2003 was hot. We all spend far too many hours in beer gardens and throwing countless barbeque parties. It really was a fantastic summer. At that point, I was only working part-time and travelling to and from Langley to labour on the roads with another friend of mine, Pete. Andy was so much fun to be around, but our livers were screaming out to us all by the autumn. Thankfully, for all of our sakes, Andy moved back to Cardiff and Sian and I moved to our first home on the Ridge! We would keep in touch. That was a certainty.

Anyway, I digress. We were going to meet Kate for the first time. Andy had recently met her following his recent separation with his wife. Kate turned out to be an amazing, lovely lady and we were all chuffed to bits for Andy. We all had a great weekend, but I found it tough to keep going and was bloody knackered for days afterwards. The rest of the month is spent much as before. Ground hogging! Walking, exercising, listening to upbeat music, lots of reading and most importantly, trying to build bridges with Sian. I know that there is a long bumpy road ahead for me as I need to regain trust and earn forgiveness for the years of constant shit I have given her over the years before finally leaving her to live in the sun without her! My crazy, depressed mind really thought it was a brilliant idea. I am willing to do whatever it takes to make Sian happy again and be the fun, outgoing person she was before my illness knocked it out of her. I am determined to have that 'Sian' back and I won't stop until I succeed.

Hey, you demon! You are not going to win anymore.
I've had it with you once and for all.
You've destroyed two people with your evil deeds.
I'm fucking coming for you now. Don't stand in my way.
I will crush you under my loafered foot!

Chapter Seven

My Experience Since Reuniting with My Husband by Sian Green

Hanging in There

I'll be honest. When Phil left, I was completely destroyed and deeply upset that after everything we had been through, our marriage had failed. Sadly, I did feel like a lead weight had been physically removed from my shoulders, my head cleared and the unending churning anxiety fell away. I soon realised that living with Phil's depression, resentment and disconnection had left me in a permanent state of fear and trepidation. Something I hadn't realised until he left and calmness flooded back into my body.

There is a mountain of information out there of ways you can help and support the person who has depression with very little regarding coping yourself as a carer. I use the word carer because I felt that's what I had become. Not a wife, lover, friend or companion but an unpaid, unhappy, sad and lonely carer who was regularly treated unfairly despite every effort to maintain the status quo at home and work. I don't feel it's unfair to admit that I felt relief once Phil had left as years of treading on eggshells and second-guessing his next move was physically exhausting and mentally crushing.

My own fault in many respects, as I hadn't set boundaries, I kept quiet when I should have spoken up, I forgave repeatedly and accepted my life for the existence it had become. More cracks began to appear as age-related changes crept up on me and the symptoms snowballed out of all proportion due to the huge stress, we were under. I did not recognise myself anymore, I had become miserable, short-tempered and quite honestly, difficult to be around. I do, however, feel annoyed and angry that I had remained in and allowed the situation to become as destructive as it had. I suppose I had put my happiness aside because in my mind, Phil was ill and I should stand by him no matter what his depression threw at us. Imagine then, after years of misplaced loyalty, my complete devastation when Phil coldly announced he was leaving for Spain.

Once Phil had finally left our home, settling into my new life was strange and lonely, yet peaceful. I did feel as if I was floating in a weird dreamlike state, carrying on with my usual routines but acutely aware of the emptiness surrounding me. I managed each day as best as I could and made an effort to see friends or pop to the gym. Everyone commented on how well I seemed but my smiling, laughing face masked the pain I was enduring inside.

Out of the blue, I started to receive the odd message from Phil, slowly expressing his change of heart and regret. Eventually, he admitted he had made a mistake and would like to come home. I agreed to talk and came to the decision to slowly try again with the understanding that we could not continue as we had left off.

Phil stayed with his brother for a few more days to organise his return which gave me time to mull over what was happening. I found myself questioning his motives and even before his return home, began to feel controlled by fear of the past repeating itself. I quickly took hold of these fears and realised that if we were to have any chance of survival, I needed to move on and forgive Phil completely. My promise was to not forget the past but I would learn from it and absolutely not repeat the mistakes I had previously made. I realised we would have bumps in the road and would make allowances for them, but there would be no return from future absolute car crashes.

Initially, I felt that Phil and I were trundling along fairly well. Phil was working again, but I soon began to notice the old patterns of abstinence remerging. I worried about the holiday I had booked and his promise of contributing towards it. We had already had a couple of short UK breaks which had been amazing. I thought the depression was under control and Phil was finally feeling a chink of happiness. The trouble with Phil is his ability to pretend, hide, deny and even lie to preserve his perception of normality. A habit he has learned over many years and will find difficult to change but change he must if we are to survive. The other problem he has is my uncanny ability to recognise these misgivings, which unfortunately do not help in rebuilding a trusting, honest relationship.

Before leaving for Greece, Phil had worked less and less and needed to use the money he had saved to pay his car rental. I could feel panic trickle back into my brain as history repeated itself. The only saving grace was that emotionally, I felt we were probably the most together we had ever been and

I could sense Phil's conscious effort to make amends. We would go to Greece, have a fabulous break and take it from there, once home and back to reality!

I could sense the fall before it happened. October came and Phil crashed spectacularly. This was it now, make or break for him, for me and for us. It was apparent that going to work was out of the question for a while and after a few weeks of R and R, I noticed an improvement in his mood. Phil actively sought help in the form of self-help books and attacking the gym more than usual. One particular book laid bare an action plan in the form of written logs, vitamin supplements, light therapy and exercise, which Phil grabbed with both hands and has pretty much followed to the letter.

I think Phil had reached the point where he was sick of just coping and wanted to be well again. He spoke to his GP practice and made an appointment to see lovely Margaret again, his mental health nurse of many years, who herself had been away ill for almost a year. Margaret put us in contact with a lottery-funded organisation who provide counselling as I was also struggling with historic issues and felt that couples counselling may be useful. Unfortunately, but realistically, the lady we saw there decided that Phil needed sole counselling before he could even contemplate dealing with our joint issues. I also organised for him to have massages with a recently found friend who is very spiritual and I trusted. During one of her visits, Phil had opened up to her and she suggested he wrote a book about his life. Again, Phil took this idea and ran with it. He has found writing about his experiences difficult at times but it has been extremely cathartic.

The wheels of the recovery bus are finally in motion and I am beginning to feel more positive about his future. However, I do feel that I'm sitting on the edge looking in; whilst Phil recovers and I continue to wait and struggle.

I say 'his' future as my demons are still very much alive and regularly remind me that we may or may not have a long journey ahead. There have been a few bumps since Phil's return, which have mirrored past episodes of vile anger and viscous hatefulness towards me. During and after these occasions, my mind replays every old, bad memory like a film on a loop and I can physically feel my brain shutting down probably in an effort to protect myself from more stress and pain. Then later, when the mist clears, questions of Phil's sincerity and candidness roll around my head and I can't find the answers. I have faith that he is doing all he can to prove he loves me, but is it real? Is Phil's mind in the here and now or is he manipulating me for his own end? Sadly, this is where I am at the moment.

The problems I have now are a result of having loved and cared for someone whose mind was fogged, unclear and confused which led to resentment, betrayal and total disconnection toward me. So many horrible events over so many years have chipped away at my heart and soul leaving me untrusting on edge and waiting for the old version of Phil to revisit.

I can say that I believe Phil's mind is much clearer now and he seems to think precisely and honestly which is what I hold onto. My absolute cornerstone to hanging in there is that Phil's attempts at rebuilding our relationship are honest, genuine and with clarity.

Chapter Eight

The Truth Hits the Heart

The truthful and totally heartfelt written account of my illness as accurately retold by my beautiful wife Sian absolutely hits me like a thunderbolt from the blue. The words I was reading I had heard before and had registered, but seeing the words written down, staring at me then hitting my brain took me by total surprise. I was knocked off guard, completely poleaxed.

I continued reading Sian's pain poured onto the paper and I began to experience that familiar aching, sickly feeling in my stomach. I didn't recognise myself as the person she was writing about. I must be someone else, not her husband and soulmate. There were some references I did recognise, including anger issues, how I shut down from people and took to my bed but there were several points I was completely unaware of and it really hurt to think that I had put Sian through so much torture and pain. Sian is right when she says that depression is no excuse to treat the one person that loves you unconditionally with a complete lack of respect and display a lack of gratitude for all she tries to do for you in your personal battle.

As I've said, this couldn't be me she was talking about, could it? When my depression hits and I become selfish, cold and unfeeling, this is definitely not the person I normally see myself as. When these words are written about you it leaves a bitter taste in your mouth with a shameful feeling. This is how this horrible illness affects me and others around me. I was completely unaware that I behave like this and I hate this illness for having the ability to turn me from a nice guy into a monster that turns on Sian in the way I do.

I feel very ashamed of myself. Leave us alone. We deserve better.

The words that hit home the hardest and left me confused and disturbed were 'despise, resent and hate.' I believe Sian 100% when she says she felt resented, despised and hated during my periods of severe depression because I probably did behave this way, it's just that I can't recall these valid points that she makes. Some people reading this might have great difficulty believing me when I say I don't remember but it's the God's honest truth. I would not behave in this manner when not afflicted by my dark demon. I love Sian with all my heart, more than I'm ever able to express to her. This illness can make you appear cold and aloof, but my feelings for her remain as strong now as they have ever been, I think stronger actually.

As far as resentment goes, that could never be attributed to Sian, in fact, she would have every right to totally resent me. What a fucking pain in the arse I am when I get depressed and I'm lower than a snake's belly. What an ungrateful sod I must come across as she would be well within her rights to not waste another moment of her life doing anything for me.

Fucking Loser

As for the word hate, I'm not even going to put that in the same sentence with Sian. I could never hate her, in any way shape or form. Again, I believe Sian when she thinks that I feel that way towards her, but again the bastard disease puts pay to my memory on this point.

I'm feeling pretty good at this point of my long road to recovery but suffice to say, it leaves me feeling horrible and very guilty.

(Sian's piece)

I am eternally grateful to Sian for having the strength and courage to write down all the painful words in the account you have just read. She is such a strong and compassionate lady and I'm so lucky to still have her by my side despite all the shit I have put her through. I am not sure where her endurance comes from. We have suffered numerous dark episodes together but have incredibly managed to come out the other side. She has always been there for me, a loving and supportive rock. I do realise that I am lucky as I'm sure most wives would have walked and I for one would not have blamed them.

Thank you, Sian, I love you so much.

We both felt we would include Sian's first-hand experiences of living with someone with depression as we felt that although the subject of mental health is slowly coming to the fore, there is little or no support for the carers. In our small way, we wanted to highlight this issue and bring awareness to the limited resources available to families and friends of people suffering from mental health problems.

Chapter Nine

No Plane to Spain

I had not noticed initially but Sian had observed a change in me from around the beginning of 2017. It wasn't uncommon for me to suffer the blues come the New Year and it is something many people experience with the onset of winter and dark days. I presumed it was just one of my usual episodes but Sian knew otherwise. I have to remind you that my illness distorts reality and I am prone to memory losses. I put that down to my brain shutting down as a kind of defence mechanism. I don't know for sure but it definitely occurs and is extremely frustrating when I attempt to recall events and facts.

I do remember feeling edgy and restless, my concentration was shot to pieces and I found it incredibly difficult to regain my thread particularly when reading. I sought solace in convincing myself that it was an age thing, so not to worry too much. Something was obviously awry, but I was blissfully unaware that this instalment was the dawning of the upcoming meltdown. The engine had started and was ticking over but I was certainly not to be the driver of this fucking monster.

On the subject of driving, I was finding it increasingly difficult to work as I could not function at the highest standards, I have always set myself. Sometimes, these levels were quite unobtainable but I strived to reach them, nonetheless. I've always taken pride in any work I've ever had but over the years, I lost interest and found it hard to get motivated in the mornings.

At the time of my meltdown, I was working as a self-employed cab driver/chauffeur which I had been enjoying. It gave me the flexibility I needed to work and could jump in and out of my car when I wanted and more importantly when I was able! Even during a relatively emotionally stable year, I would have at least a couple of depressive episodes rendering me unable to work for up to a couple of weeks. I was able to take time off when I needed and without having to explain this invisible illness to an employer.

This scenario worked well for several years until the meltdown monster kicked into second gear. I was beginning to let work down more and more. I would cancel the advance bookings I had previously accepted, on occasions hours before I was due to collect my fare. This was not me whatsoever.

What's wrong with you, Phil? You don't do this, you're reliable.

Get a fucking grip, will you?

The truth of the matter was that although I would make the excuse that I was ill, I really was. I just wasn't aware of it at the time. I was always able to communicate well with my passengers. A bit of banter, a mundane discussion about the weather or just lending an ear for problems people seemed willing to share with me. I loved picking up the 'oldies' as they always had a story, funny tale or rude joke to tell. I picked up two lovely ladies, who were 101 and 103 years old. They were amazing, both mobile and doing their own shopping and neither looked anywhere near their ages. Bloody brilliant! Anyway, I digress.

I started to withdraw more and more towards my passengers. I used to begin conversations, but it soon became the job of my clients. Looking back, this was another sign that I was probably spending my waking hours away with the fairies. Previously, my passengers had always expressed how lovely it was to have a polite, chatty driver who had made their journey a pleasant one. I dreaded the longer journeys as I found it so hard to engage with anyone.

How mad is that? What is happening to my head? Will someone please help me?

Obviously, I was struggling with so many things at that time but try as I might remember, I cannot recall a couple of months leading up to Sian's 50th birthday. I'm almost sure by this time that I had suffered my second major depressive episode of the year along with many mini dips that eventually lead me to not work completely. I felt terrible and extremely guilty as I really wanted to do something special to mark the occasion of Sian's birthday. Two years ago, Sian had taken me to Benidorm for my 50th birthday with another ten friends and had a bloody fantastic time and I wanted the same for her. The problem was that I was not working regularly enough beforehand and couldn't save the necessary funds. I felt bloody rotten.

This fucking illness! Why won't you let me feel normal?

I want Sian to have the best. If me being afflicted wasn't now Sian is the one who's going to suffer. Fuck you!

As Sian has mentioned in her piece, not very long after her birthday, I made the announcement that I wanted to get away and live in Spain. In my depressed, addled mind, this felt like the best option for me. My father and a couple we both knew had moved to Spain in their 50s and it seemed a perfectly good and logical thing to do. I was in my 50s and had spent many holidays in Spain enjoying the sun and a relaxed pace. Sian and I had holidayed in the area that our friends, Byron and Donna had moved to and also stayed with them the year before. With all this in mind, I came to the conclusion that this would be the perfect area for me to start a new life. As I'm writing this now, it seems crazy but at the time I was convinced that this was what I wanted. I spoke with Byron and asked him to look for available villas to rent and he came back to me saying that a friend wanted a long-term tenant. Perfect I thought.

Whilst preparing to leave and making the necessary arrangements, I carried on living at home with Sian. It was a difficult period but we both tried really hard to be civil to each other. Obviously, things were not great and the atmosphere was somewhat strained. Sian was amazing at sorting out the various aspects of separating including the finances, solicitor and even the packing. She was and is always absolutely brilliant. What was I thinking? I was even showing her pictures of the villas when inside she's dying. I didn't realise the hurt I was causing. To my depressed mind, all this is normal and as it should be. The meltdown monster is almost ready to shift up into third gear, I think.

Why can't I see what I'm doing to Sian? You're throwing everything away, you idiot!

The demon in my head is laughing to himself. You evil bastard!

Towards the end, Sian was leaving the house as much as possible because it was too painful for her to be around me. I'm still blissfully unaware of the hurt I'm causing her but when I look back now, it's bloody obvious. This is the strength and power that severe depression holds over you. Eventually, Sian can take it no longer and asks me to move out. I knew it couldn't carry on, it was unworkable and I agreed. One phone call later and it's off to Slough I go.

I texted my brother, Rich and I asked him if it was okay to stay for a short while. It would probably be only four weeks or so before I could leave for Spain. Thankfully, he agreed but I had to wait a week because his girlfriend and kids had popped over from Ireland to visit. This wasn't a major problem but it meant that Sian had another week of going out to avoid being around me. The week came and went fairly quickly, which was probably a blessing.

Sian helped me load the car with basically just the clothes I would need for Spain and a few sets of weights so I was able to train whenever possible. Sian agreed to store my remaining possessions in the garage.

See what I mean, Sian is always brilliant!

Why am I walking away from all this?

Of course, the above statements don't enter a depressed foggy head. Although I'm a million miles away in cloud cuckoo land, I'm lucid enough to realise that I'm not feeling very good and heavy-hearted. Pangs of guilt hit me hard and I just don't know what to say on the journey down to my brothers. How crazy is that? Here was somebody I'd known since I was sixteen years old, she was my soulmate, best friend and more importantly, she was still my wife. She might as well have been a complete stranger to me, just a driver who had the good grace to pick me up as if I was hitchhiking.

The journey to Slough seemed to take much longer than usual. I've no doubt that Sian felt the same and we were both relieved when we finally arrived at Richards gaff. Sian has since told me that all said to her was "thanks for the lift" as I turned and walked away. Not a sorry or thank you for the past fifteen years. I just couldn't find the right words and probably thought that whatever I said was not going to make the situation any better for either of us. Looking back now with a clearer head, I wish I had said something to Sian. It was the least she deserved and I would like to apologise to Sian for my total lack of feeling.

I'm So Sorry Sian X

It was true that I walked off but once she had driven off, I walked to the end of the road and watched as Sian disappeared into the distance. That was a surreal feeling. When I said I was off to Slough, I actually meant Langley where Sian and I both

42

grew up and originally met. Some people refer to Langley as near Windsor but actually it bangs next door to Slough. But that's another story!

I was extremely grateful to Rich for putting me up at very short notice because I was basically in the shit street. Many thanks, bruv. After the first days at my brother's, I felt lighter. Perhaps because the pressure had lifted as Sian and I had some distance between us. Don't get me wrong, I still felt bloody rotten over the whole situation and my head felt completely washed out. I can only imagine how Sian was feeling but probably not great! I attempt to train, but I'm not enjoying it. On the upside, Rich and I get to spend some time together. We go out for a few enjoyable bevvies on occasion like a pair of old farts putting the world to rights. Most days were spent on my own giving me unlimited time to mull over my thoughts, which is not a good thing when I'm not feeling my best.

Over the course of the first week, I tried to align my thoughts which was proving a complete waste of time. The more I ruminated the more confusing my mind became. Sian and I agreed that I should not contact her unless it was in an emergency, but there were times when I wanted to call for advice and to check she was ok. However, I respected her wishes on that front and kept away. I had already spoken to Byron's friend about the villa, which was not available until the end of August, which wasn't a problem as Rich had already said I could stay as long as I needed.

There was a problem brewing. Toward the end of the second week, I began to have doubts in my mind regarding going to Spain. Not because I didn't want to go to Spain, but because I didn't want to do it without Sian. I was really missing her and I took the decision to ignore her wishes and contact her. First, I asked if she was okay then I started to tell her of my doubts that were creeping in more and more. We eventually spoke on the phone and decided to meet up for a talk to try and resolve everything. Sian agreed I could come home again with a few conditions attached. I informed Rich of my decision and again thanked him for all he had done for me in my hour of need. Thanks again, Rich.

While all this was going on, I still felt way under par. The meltdown monster was still in third gear and taking his time but his mate, the evil little demon seemed to be on holiday. I wasn't experiencing many episodes of ruminating, but my mood was still subdued. I attempted to go back to work in the weeks before we were due to go on holiday to Greece. It was okay, but I was still finding it harder than usual to function normally. Sian and I seem to be getting on well but hey ho, there's a lot of work still ahead of us. I had already informed Byron's friend that I now didn't want to take her offer of the villa.

Our holiday in Greece was fantastic. Sunny, hot and beautiful every single day while considering it was late September and coming to the end of the holiday season. We really couldn't have expected any more. We both temporarily forgot our problems and just soaked up the sun. My mood always picks up when the sun is shining, it really does. Maybe my demon is on holiday too as he's not made himself known to me. Who knows?

I know now, however, that he was on a break, gathering his power and strength for my return home before he could finally take me down properly in a few weeks' time.

The Little Fucker!

The holiday played out perfectly. We really did have an amazing time in Greece. The country is stunning, the food gorgeous, the people are lovely and the cocktails fantastic. We both loved it. We returned home and settled into a normal life. Sian returned to work and I started to hit the road again. It didn't take me very long to become aware that the demon was waking from his slumber once more. The meltdown monster hits fourth gear. Negative thoughts and the churning stomach, here we go again. I knew it was coming. I'm never sure when it's going to arrive but when it does, it's quick and completely at its mercy. The black cloud of doom descends upon me like a heavy, giant blanket totally enveloping me. I feel helpless, unable to function and I crawl into bed.

I'm Fucked!

As was so often the case, several days later and I resurface. A few days later and I return to work but looking back now, it was too soon. I was trying so hard because apart from needing the money, I wanted our relationship to work and to show Sian that I was deadly serious about our relationship. I knew I was in a bad place, but I felt that I had to carry on for Sian's sake and mine. I was starting to miss days of work again. I just couldn't build a head of steam no matter how hard I tried. I felt I was letting my bosses down but more importantly I was letting Sian down, but as hard as I tried, it was a complete and utter futile struggle.

More days in bed followed and this was my first real inkling that I was not just ill with my normal episode of depression. I had not had close and recurrent depressive episodes before. This was new to me. I was so worried for so many reasons. Worried that Sian would finally have had enough of me and my illness, worried that this was moving to another level and finally kill me. I was so unsure, concerned and bloody frightened.

The demons laughing at me again! I'm finally beating you at long last. Give up. You've lost the war.

The meltdown monster hits top gear.

He was right. By now, it's early October. What day, hour or minute it couldn't say, but it finally happened. It hits home and wipes me out. This is the final battle of the war and I don't know if I'm going to come back in one piece.

Only time will tell!

Chapter Ten

S.T.C.

December arrived; it was now the countdown to Christmas. I was dreading the event and just wanted the whole thing to disappear under a huge rock. It was going to be the first time in my 35 years working life that I would have no funds to spend on presents or fun. Sian and I don't generally go mad spending wise when it comes to gifts but we would normally but two or three small items, these would be opened on Christmas morning along with our champagne and bacon butties. Sian had already mentioned that we shouldn't worry about buying presents for each other that year and that I was not to worry myself over the matter. But hey, that's what everybody says under those circumstances, isn't it?

As the days passed through, I was beginning to feel very guilty about the situation. I was used to having money to spend, this was all alien to me and I felt really bad about this. The word 'sponger' used to cross my mind quite often, I just couldn't help it. Of course, I knew that it wasn't the most important thing in the world if I couldn't buy Sian any gifts, it was more important that we had each other and had good health, even if I didn't completely have mine! I'd taken in what Sian had said, but my depressed jumbled up head just wasn't getting it. Being married is being part of a team and it's probably very common for one half of that team to be unable to work at some point, so why was I feeling so guilty? The fact that I was only functioning at about 50/60% at the time might have had something to do with it, this was a small improvement from November, but still a long way from what I considered to be normal.

The only counting down I was actively doing at that time was counting down the days that I could secure an appointment with Margaret Corcoran. I really was treading water, not making any significant progress in my battle with the illness and all the anti-depressant pill-popping in the world just wasn't enough for me any longer. I needed professional help and quick! Groundhog Day continued, my reading of books has picked up, I seem to be reading them twice as quickly as before. A certain online retailer must be starting to love me! When the weather permitted, I did my walking and I worked out regularly also but I was finding it hard to find enough energy to make the sessions beneficial. It felt like I was on a treadmill of limbo, just existing, not living a full and satisfying life. I know Sian felt the same too. It's hard writing these words some five months later to imagine what it was really like to live with me, it must have been torture I'm sure. I remember very little of this time now if I'm brutally honest, it's all a hazy blur and makes me feel very rubbish. My mind was in self-preservation mode, making me appear cold and uncaring towards Sian, but I was doing enough to keep me going, surviving another day, a necessary act almost.

As the days edged towards Christmas, I still had pangs of guilt.

Get over yourself, you muppet.

Head, give me a break, will ya?

I'm so tired of this now

Close to Christmas, we'd arranged to visit my mum and Dave in Colnbrook because we were not going to be seeing them over the holidays. Looking back, I can't recall the trip very much, most of it escapes me now, how bad is that? God knows what my poor mum thought. I must have been someone she barely recognised. I felt sad and ashamed in equal measure, I just hope I didn't upset her too much, sorry Mum x.

I received an early Christmas present, I'd managed to arrange an appointment with Margaret, it was booked for five days before Christmas and I was really looking forward to seeing her once again. Deep down, I was really hoping that this was going to get the ball rolling and start the process of my recovery. At the appointment, I explained every detail to Margaret about what had happened in October, my breakdown and how it had badly affected me and Sian. I finished off by describing how the whole year had been very traumatic and upsetting and that we were both at our wit's end. Margaret suggested that she could refer us to an organisation named SWADS for couples counselling, we both agreed straight away, so Margaret made the call and an appointment was arranged for the 3 January 2018.

Christmas day duly arrived and I wasn't too sure how it was going to pan out. Sian had purchased some bottles of 'bubbles', so we had our customary few glasses with our breakfast, all very nice. We opened presents we'd received from the family and of course from my stepdaughter, Becky.

It felt a bit strange not opening a gift from Sian, but it wasn't as bad as I was expecting. Lunchtime was spent in one of our nearby pubs with Emma and John, some very good friends of ours and then we both enjoyed a relatively quiet afternoon/evening slobbed out in front of the TV watching Christmas repeats. We have a tradition on Boxing Day whereby we meet up with friends in the local pub. This 'sesh' normally starts up at lunchtime, just in time for all the great Boxing Day footy that is on the box, it really is my favourite day of the year. Under normal circumstances, we would all then pile around somebody's gaff for more drinks and copious amounts of food but Sian and myself were not really 'feeling it' and so we decided to head home early evening and have a quiet night. This summed up our Christmas, very understated by our normal standards.

I know that both of us were relieved that we'd managed to get through Christmas unscathed. We tried hard to have a good time, but we were both mentally scarred by the recent events and our enthusiasm for the festivities just wasn't there. The most defining detail regarding this particular Christmas and the one thing that I hadn't even realised until the festive season was over was the fact that I hadn't even heard my favourite seasonal tune, S.T.C. This epitomised Christmas 2017, but it was appropriate in some small way because I decided to use the song title for the heading of this chapter.

New Year approached and for as long as I can remember, we would always go out on New Year's Eve. It's Sian's favourite night of the year. A good barometer as to measure how Sian wasn't 'feeling it' would be to tell you that she simply couldn't be bothered to go out. We were so glad to see the back of 2017, it had been a terrible year, but equally, both of us were also feeling very apprehensive about what the New Year might possibly bring us. We both hoped that 2018 would be much better. But until I managed to get some much-needed help, we were both on an emotional treadmill trip to nowhere and we couldn't wait to get off!

The ball had been set in motion
There was a chink of light finally
Could I dare to hope?
Could I lay bare my soul?

Chapter Eleven

Blues and Soul – Part 1

Sian and I made the short trip into town on that first Wednesday in January 2018. We were visiting SWADS, an organisation that Margaret had referred us to. It had initially been set up to help people with drink and drug problems but had branched out into the mental health sector. It is a charitable enterprise helped by donations and happens to be funded by a large lottery company. To help with the growing needs of local people living with mental health problems, the organisation is currently in the process of expansion. This involves employing more counsellors, a positive sign of all the good work that they do.

I rang the bell on that door for the first time, a small action I'd repeat many times in the ensuing months ahead. We were met by a lovely lady called Barbara who welcomed us in. I went on to explain in detail my whole mental health history, the suicide attempts and how my destructive illness had impacted on Sian throughout the whole time of my battle with the dark side. Barbara pointed out that they also offered other 'alternative therapies' which included music and art classes. I must admit to being slightly sceptical as to how that would benefit me to be totally honest, I mean I'm crap at drawing and as much as I love my music, my playing skills stretched to playing the triangle at primary school! I said that I'd give the matter some thought, however, what I needed more at that time was 'heavy therapy' that was going to be my total priority.

The initial thinking was that Sian and I would have couples counselling, but Barbara insisted that I should have one to one session to begin with. I needed to get 'fixed' first before we could think about taking on sessions together, so a unanimous verdict was reached, I would be flying solo. Barbara stated that she'd be in touch very soon with an appointment and I left that building with a renewed sense of vigour. I was absolutely determined that I was going to grab the opportunity with both hands and nothing and no one was going to get in my way. Within a day or two, Barbara called me, my first appointment was arranged for Wednesday 24 January, she wished me good luck and said that she was always at the other end of the phone if I ever needed any help whatsoever.

As I drove into town on that fateful day, I was feeling extremely nervous at the prospect of my first counselling session. A lady by the name of Isobel was awaiting me, but I wasn't nervous at the thought of meeting her, I'd got used to meeting new people on a daily basis when working as a cabbie/chauffeur, but I was well aware that this was a watershed moment for me. The importance of the start of that process cannot be understated, this was going to be 'shit or bust'. There was no coming back from this point. The obvious reasons why this had to work didn't need spelling out, if it didn't work, it could spell the end of mine and Sian's relationship, it really was that important.

For the very first time in my fifty-two years, I was about to lay bare my heart, my soul and all of the grisly details that had afflicted me for so long. People that know me will no doubt be shocked by what they read, I'm not going to hold anything back, if I'm ever to get better and make a full recovery, it all needs to come out. I knock on the door of SWADS, this was going to be a defining moment in my life, one I'm certain I will never forget.

Session 1

The door opened, the lady standing before me introduced herself as Natalie. She welcomed me inside and asked me to take my place in the waiting room. Isobel would be with me very shortly I was told. The butterflies in my stomach were fluttering around like crazy as I took my seat on a comfy leather chair. Located next to me was a tropical fish tank, the fish were swimming around without a care in the world and for a few seconds, I had the thought that it must be nice to be a fish, living a peaceful existence and not having personal problems to worry about. All of this was a million miles away from what I was about to subject myself to and for those few seconds the goldfish's life seemed more preferable to mine.

Before I knew it, another lady popped her head around the door and introduced herself as Isobel, she was my counsellor. I followed her down a narrow hallway until we came to a door, a door that opened up to an unremarkable room, a room where I would lay bare my soul, my strengths, my weaknesses, in fact, my whole life to who was technically a total stranger (sorry Isobel). My nerves had started to subside just a little bit, Isobel's kind demeanour had begun to put me at ease and I felt that I was going to be relatively comfortable with telling her everything, warts and all about my mental health issues.

This first session was to be more of an overview, she had to learn from me all about my history, i.e. when my mental health problems started, what had triggered them, what I'd done in the past to tackle them, was I on medication. She had to build up a picture of me quickly, which was never going to be an easy task, considering the long battle I'd had with my depression. I started off by telling Isobel that I'd been adopted as a baby and it was a fact, I'd been aware of since I was very young. My 'Mum' had never tried to hide the fact, she had always been upfront with me about it. I stated that being adopted had never been a problem for me and didn't think it had contributed to my depression. We spoke at great length about my illness, I said that I was convinced that my depression had manifested itself when I was around seventeen, not at the extreme levels that have afflicted me in recent years, but I became aware of its existence.

Isobel then asked me if I knew any specific reasons as to why my depression had started. I remember pausing for a few seconds (this was it, the point of no return, Phil). I've got several 'I said' but some are more relevant than others. "I was bullied at school but I would be happy to leave that to next time if that's okay?"

"No problem, Phil." (This was it, what I was about to reveal may cause some shockwaves amongst some people.)

My dad sexually abused me! Just five small words that encapsulated over forty years of mental suffering. My family had never known my terrible secret, but I had to get this heavy rock off my chest once and for all. I was to do this one night after consuming many drinks (I needed a lot of Dutch courage). This was going to be very difficult for me. I felt the best way was to tell my three brothers by way of a text message, at least I wouldn't have to face them when they learnt of my horrific disclosure. There was never going to be an easy or right way of telling my family about the abuse, but I felt happy that I'd finally exorcised the ghost of abuse by getting it out there, it was a massive relief for me. Days, months and years of excruciating soul searching on my part had got me to this point but this was just the start. As I write this now, the subject of abuse has never been raised by anybody in my family, my brothers included. I do understand the many reasons why this is so and I don't blame them at all. The sexual abuse had taken place four decades earlier and I still feel no good will come of it by dragging it up anymore, after all, I was now dealing with the demon and at the end of the day, it was my battle.

Isobel is a very calm person and I wasn't sure how she'd taken my confession at first, to be honest. I mean, just how do you react when that is put to you? "I'm so sorry," Isobel said, "Would you like to talk about it, Phil?"

I paused for a short time before answering, I was trying to make sure I had my facts straight in my head, after all, it was a very long time ago. I said to Isobel that I was around nine or ten years of age, I was living in Langley at the time (where I grew up) and my parents had separated at that point. My dad would arrive at different times to either look after us or take us out on occasions. It was at these times that the abuse took place, I can't recall how many times it actually happened, but happen it did. I explained to Isobel that I didn't want to go into graphic detail regarding the abuse, the fact that I was talking about it was enough for me. Another reason for my stance on this is that I've no desire to cause further upset to my family if they ever get to read this book.

Isobel glanced at the clock; we'd come to the end of our first of many sessions together. I was already starting to feel like that giant rock was beginning to lift off my chest, I was on my way, I'd started the process of getting well again and it felt good. Isobel thanked me for being very open with her, she knew it had been hard for me, but I left that building on Milton Road, Swindon with a spring in my step and I for one was only intending at looking in one direction, there would be no backwards glances from me from that moment on.

Session 2

I knew when I undertook these sessions that I'd probably experience some emotional fallout. This certainly happened after my first session, I was very tired and physically drained for a couple of days afterwards. It was fairly obvious, it had to go hand in hand, I'd started to release all of my emotional baggage, baggage that I'd carried on my person for over four decades. I was well aware that I had to roll with the punches, it was never going to be easy and to think otherwise would have been naive on my part. For some reason, a nagging thought kept entering my head concerning my disclosure of my sexual abuse, had I done the right thing? I knew all of the potential ramifications of my bringing out into the open the incident of sexual abuse, but I was also aware that it had to come out of the box, it was just too important to be swept under the carpet.

I arrived at Bradford House for my second session with Isobel, I still had some nerves for some strange reason, but once Isobel greeted me with her nice warm smile, I immediately felt at ease. A warm feeling suddenly enveloped me and I knew everything was going to be ok. We both sat down and I was asked if I was ok. How was I feeling? How had the last week been? I began to tell Isobel that although it had been good to talk about my abuse, it had left its mark on me. I was feeling mentally and physically tired even a week on from our first session. I explained further about the nagging thoughts that kept entering my head in relation to the abuse I'd suffered at the hands of my dad. "Do you think you did the right thing, Phil?" Isobel asked.

I said, "Yes! Definitely, I do." I felt that I needed to explain that although the nagging thoughts were still there under the surface, they had actually started to subside and upon reflection, I'd taken the right course of action. "Are you happy to leave the subject of abuse now" Isobel enquired.

I said, "Yeah, I'm happy to leave it there for now thanks."

"Before we leave this behind, Phil, I'd like to know your thoughts about the fact your family has never brought the subject of abuse up with you?" It wasn't an easy question to answer straight away.

"I suspect that it must have come as a massive shock to them, I mean just where do you start when trying to get your head around that I exclaimed!" As I've already said, I don't blame my brothers one bit for not wanting to broach the subject with me. They'd grown up with an image of their father and I'd shattered that picture in one text message! That revelation would blow most people's world apart and I really don't want to subject them or my mum in particular to any more hurt and upset. I finished off by asking Isobel if she thought I was being selfish for letting this proverbial cat out of the bag?

"What do you mean, Phil?"

"I mean the fact I was revealing all of this horror, purely in the hope of making myself feel better."

"Of course not, Phil," Isobel replied. I said I just wanted to let sleeping dogs lie and asked if we could move on, please?

"What would you like to cover next" Isobel enquired.

"I would like to talk about the bullying I suffered at school." I never realised until now that talking so much makes you incredibly thirsty (for people that don't know me, I feel it needs to be said that I'm not the world's biggest talker), a sip from my glass was needed. It was explained to Isobel that I'd attended the worst school in Slough, its reputation was justly earned. Academically, I gave up. It was only sports such as football and cricket that I was seriously interested in and to a lesser degree, I also took part in basketball and athletics. I played for all of the above school teams, it was the only reason I bothered turning up for school most days, the other days I 'wagged'. This school was called Holmewood, it's long since gone but its fearsome reputation still lives on.

"My first year at this school was the most traumatic," I told Isobel, "the bullying was terrible." At that young age, some aspects of life escape you, you are naive, lack experience and don't always see things as they really are. My best mate at the time had two older brothers, who also attended Holmewood, they had a reputation for looking after themselves, so through no fault of his own, my best mate got left alone. My problem, I explained to Isobel, was I got associated with their 'little brother', so I got picked on. At that time, it didn't cross my mind (what with being a wet behind the ears first-year grunt) that this was the reason for my problems. It wasn't my mate's fault really and the punches around the head, the kicks up the arse would occur when he was not in my presence so he never knew and I've never told him to this day.

I explained to Isobel that you couldn't take liberties at that school otherwise you'd get a 'clump around the ear' for your troubles. I would get to feel this on numerous occasions often for no apparent reason other than making the perpetrator laugh! In the end, I used to dread the thought of school the following day, I would lie in bed feeling physically sick, knowing for sure I'd get a kicking or sometimes something worse. The only times I looked forward to attending was if there was a games lesson or a match after school, other than that, I couldn't face my bullies, they were killing my self-esteem on a daily basis. I had numerous days 'sick' where I would lie to my mum, saying I was ill or any excuse that I could come up with, not facing my bullies even for one day would be a blessed relief!

I somehow managed to get through that first year at Holmewood and that summer came as a massive respite for me, six weeks where hopefully I'd be left alone and not receive a 'ten-hole Doc Marten boot up my arse!'

Unfortunately for me, even though the passage of time passes much slower when you're a kid, the six weeks soon passed. The week leading up to my return and my subsequent second year found me experiencing feelings of anxiety and I just felt sick inside. I really didn't want to face my tormentors once again, but I had no choice in the matter. The second year started, but I seemed to be no longer their priority for a 'daily clump!' I'm not saying that the bullying stopped completely because it didn't, but it was explained to Isobel that generally, my second year was a lot better overall.

That said that was until one day my services were required as a goalkeeper for the above year football team. They had an important match and for reasons that escape me now, they had no goalkeeper. It was a position I'd played in since I was roughly eight or nine years of age playing for my local youth team. At that time, it needs to be explained that I was a right scrawny so and so, legs like two pieces of cotton (you get the picture) and potentially getting injured against bigger lads was not a predicament I wanted as it would mean missing the game at the weekend. I believe I was approached by my games teacher who asked me if I could help out the older lads by playing the game. I expressed my reservations and he replied, "fair enough" and I thought that was the end of the matter.

This was to be a naive mistake on my part, the following day I was making my way across the playground towards the gym when suddenly I was pounced on by four or five lads who were part of the football team, two of them just happened to be my main tormentors. They basically told me I had to play or I'd get a 'kicking'. I replied, "No, I ain't, fuck off, you can't make me play you 'c***s!'." Obviously, it was another mistake I made because the next thing that happened to me was that I was bundled to the ground by my perpetrators, who each grabbed one of my limbs. I can more than look after myself but I had no chance fending off these bullies and to my horror, I found that I was being carried towards the gym and where I'd receive 'my punishment'. I knew exactly what was coming up, I'd witnessed some other poor souls receive this form of medieval torture sometime before and I was shit scared. Time seemed to slow down, it was all a bit surreal and no pleading on my part was going to work in changing the minds of these lads. For the record, I was about to receive 'the Holmewood posting'. I remember bracing myself for what was to come, there was no point in me struggling, this would only end up with me receiving 'more hits'.

The first excruciating blow hit home, right on my crown jewels. The pain was indescribable, I'd been kicked in the bollocks before, but the pain was another level on this occasion. What made the ordeal even worse was the fact that the posts were square in design, perfect for inflicting maximum pain and then the second blow arrived. The searing pain that shot through my body almost made me pass out, all men can attest the pain of receiving a blow in the 'gonads', this was a thousand times worse. They let me go, I hit the ground, I was pulling my legs up towards my stomach, the pain in my groin area and stomach was leaving me unable to speak, I couldn't get my words out, but finally I managed to let them know that I'd play, they had won, I was fucked.

They walked off and left me in a crumpled heap, not one person came to my aid, fearing that they'd get the same if they intervened. I explained to Isobel that that was what it was like back then, a terrible school and a totally different time in history. The game was played the following day after school and even though I was suffering from a really swollen groin, I'd managed to play a blinder. We even won the game I told Isobel and perhaps most curiously, I eventually ended up playing for all of the above year football teams!

The fact I was now playing and mixing with the older lads, resulted happily for me in that I was left alone, the bullying stopped, but unfortunately, this spawned in me a new and bad type of behaviour. I became very rebellious and perhaps most disturbing of all, I turned into a bully myself! Isobel said to me, "Why do you think that happened?"

"I'm not 100% certain, to be honest," I replied, maybe I was lashing out at everybody. The 'posting' had left an indelible mark on me; I was definitely mentally scarred by the experience, that's for sure. I told Isobel that in a warped kind of way that was probably my way of processing my hurt and anger, I had no other way of dealing with it at the time, anger was all I understood and was an easy outlet for me. Another feeling I had at the time was that I felt badly let down by the school.

"Let down," Isobel quizzed.

"Yeah, let down because of the bullying and also the fact that they weren't actively stopping me from bullying either." I was being allowed to 'work out my anger on innocent people'. I wasn't trying to hide the fact either as I did get in trouble for hitting pupils and no real punishment was ever handed out. A school is somewhere where you go to learn not a place that you should ever feel frightened to attend, so all of the bullying was wrong on every level.

Isobel paused for a few seconds before saying, "Yes, you were badly let down, Phil."

Isobel then asked me a difficult question to answer, "How long did the bullying of others continue?" I had to think long and hard, I'd never given the matter much thought, but I said that I was pretty sure that it had stopped early during my third year. That's not to say my problems had totally stopped, I was still getting in trouble quite often with my teachers because I just wasn't interested in learning. I hated that school and sport

63

was my only outlet. I stressed to Isobel that I always feel very shameful when I look back at that period when I bullied others, it is something I don't feel very proud of and a horrible feeling in the pit of my stomach is always felt by myself, even as I write this account now. Hindsight is a wonderful thing, looking back I've often wondered that things might have been better for me if I had told my peers sooner about the fact I was being bullied, but who knows if it would have made any difference back then, things were very different. I was just a kid, perhaps a product of the time, but it was still very, very wrong.

Isobel and I both glanced at the clock, another session had flown by and it had been very traumatic and emotional for me. I felt a total wreck. I knew these sessions were going to be hard, but I had no idea really just how very hard they were going to be. "See you next week," Isobel said.

"Yeah," I replied, although by this point, I was on automatic pilot, the words being spoken by both of us weren't really registering with me, I was 'shot' and had nothing left to give after that appointment at Bradford House. If I could take any consolation from my feeling like shit, it was the positive fact in my mind that I'd probably touched on the two most toughest specific reasons as to why I'd suffered the debilitating illness. That is my 'black dog'. The bitch that is depression!

Chapter Twelve
Looney Tunes

It was the second week in August and Sian and I were in the early stages of getting our relationship back up and running again. There was a music event coming up that I hadn't expected to attend as Sian and I had separated. The event was the Great Northern Ska Festival held in Manchester. Sian had bought me tickets as a present for the previous Christmas.

See what I mean! What a beautiful, lovely lady she is, so thoughtful.

I was so longing forward to going before Sian and I began having our problems, problems that I alone brought to our front door.

What a bloody idiot I am. You are a fool, Phil!
I give up, you really do take the biscuit mate.

It's fair to say that I felt gutted when it appeared that I won't be able to attend the festival. It was a present from Sian and I had absolutely no intention of going alone, it just didn't feel right. Now I was like a big kid again. I had grown up with the music and movement when the country had felt all but abandoned by the political establishment. The music was a loud reminder to the stuffed shirts in parliament that many were fed up of being ignored and trodden on. I couldn't wait to be surrounded by likeminded people who shared the same passion as me. The 2-tone explosion that rocked the foundations of this once great country arrived during the late 1970s. I was in my early teens and the first song I heard was from my future favourite 2-tone band. People say that sometimes when you first hear a piece of music, it can knock you sideways and always remember where you were at the time. I can tell you precisely. I was on a family holiday at Butlins when I heard the track and had never experienced anything like it before. The pure energy raised the hairs on the back of my neck like soldiers standing to attention. I rushed to the DJ like my life depended on it and he told me about this new band.

That was the moment my love for ska and 2-tone music was born. The Specials had black and white band members and the music proved to be a positive and powerful weapon towards easing the racist tension growing amongst young people at that time. Without getting too political, the countries unrest was why 2-tone evolved. I loved everything about it. It was infectious and you couldn't help but jump around and dance to the beat. Other bands began to spawn. All producing energetic tracks depicting the times we were living through.

The clothes worn definitely made you stand out from the crowd. The rude boys and girls had arrived donning 2-tone tonic suits worn with loafers or brogues finished with a trilby or pork pie hat. That look was so smart but you could dress down with Sta Press trousers and Fred Perry polo shirts. My particular favourite was and still is a Ben Sherman shirt, Sta Press trousers and tasselled loafers. What a look! Even now, I get positive comments and curious looks from people who can't identify with the image and catch them looking at the badges on my hat to see what they say or mean.

On the other hand, I'm not alone as recently there appears to be an emergence of many fans of the era, young and old. Social media groups sprung up regularly promoting music and fashion. Unfortunately, all too often, a huge misconception that is tagged onto the image was when the Skinheads emerged. They turned up in jeans, high Doc Marten boots, braces and Fred Perry shirts and trouble did at times escalate. You have to remember how unstable the social climate was and many forgotten young people were unemployed and angry with their desperate situation.

The day arrived, Sian and I headed up to Manchester with ska music blaring out all the way up the M6, the car was bouncing. The venue was on Trafford Park and we were staying at a hotel bang next door to Old Trafford. We settled in our room and headed off to the bar for a couple of warm-up beers. Lubrication for my poor knackered knees you understand! We jumped in a cab and arrived at the venue around 1 pm, ready for twelve hours of fun in this converted warehouse. It appeared well organised with plenty of food stands emanating gorgeous smelling grub. We were greeted by the sight of skins and rude boys and girls, which took me right back to 1979 as we entered. I was excited from the palpable buzz and energy which enthralled the building. There were two main stages at either end of the warehouse, which enabled one band to finish and another to start without annoying intervals for the full twelve hours.

There was already a large crowd gathering, people mingling and checking out the many stands selling 2 tone and ska memorabilia. I was in heaven. There were retro clothes, accessories, hats, badges and braces, the whole shabang. Perhaps more importantly, there were two large bars which were obviously expecting an extremely busy day as I spotted pallets of beer stacked high behind the temporary bars. Bloody hell, I know beer and music go together but this sight was mind-blowing. Before very long the music began, this was its knees, get ready for action! People were warming up and the dancing began in fury, bearing in mind it was still only two o'clock. The sight in front of me was surreal and incredible in equal measures. So many individuals dressed in attire that stepped back to the past. Rude boys, girls, skins and even a few mods. Just bloody brilliant, I can tell ya!

After a few beers and hours, the action stepped up a gear and although the festival is in its infancy, the bands were amazing. The organisers are keen for this to become an established, well-known event to encourage bigger acts to participate. We and many others had worked up an appetite and a food pit stop were called for and perhaps a well-earned rest. We stuck to the theme of the day and enjoyed some amazing Jamaican food. My knees were already shouting give it a rest old man. Piss off, not a chance. Sian and I had no intention of stopping, we were having such a fantastic time. The atmosphere was electric with no hint of trouble. Back in the day, there would be no way mods and skinheads could share the same air without a punch up ensuing. This was different as everybody just sucked up the experience and enjoyed each other's company. Day turned into night and the lubrication seemed to be working in as much as I couldn't feel my knees anymore. The more we jumped and danced about the more lubrication we needed. Funny that!

Time marched on and finally late into the evening, we sat on some very sticky stairs and admitted defeat along with many other poor middle-aged sods. We called a cab back to our hotel and I knew that I was physically going to pay dearly for my high jinks. I didn't care but is fair to say that we literally crawled into bed and were asleep as soon as our heads hit the pillow. The following day, my worst fears were confirmed. My knees were totally shagged, but we planned to pub crawl around Manchester which we did and, in my case, it definitely was a crawl!

Chapter Thirteen
Blues and Soul – Part 2

Session 3

From a personal point of view, session three and four were slightly less traumatic than my previous two, however, they were no less taxing on my mind and soul. The subject matter was still going to be of a heavy nature and I knew I was in for a tough time. It was the 7 February 2018 and having arrived at Bradford House, I found myself sat opposite Isobel once again in that rather unassuming room. "Hello, Phil, what would you like to get off your chest tonight?"

I decided that I wanted to discuss my first marriage. It had ended very badly with hurt, anger and a lot of bitterness on both sides. The fallout from the marriage had left me badly scarred and I explained that we'd shared twenty years together, thirteen of those married. "That's quite a long time," Isobel remarked, "Yeah, I know," I replied and we were very young when we first got together. We were married at twenty-three and I said that maybe we had 'outgrown one another'. I explained further that there were two children involved in the divorce and the whole situation had got very acrimonious, it was not something I personally wanted at any cost.

I'm now a grandad I explained and my daughter has given me two lovely granddaughters. "Congratulations, Phil," said Isobel. But I had to point out that I still hadn't been lucky enough to meet them. My relationship with my son and daughter had been somewhat fraught on one hand and non-existent on the other. I needed to pause and take a much-needed sip of water. I told Isobel that I'd only seen my daughter once in sixteen years and hadn't seen my son at all during that time.

"It had killed me," I said.

"I'm so sorry to hear that, Phil, that must have been very hard for you?" Talking about this was so hard for me, part of me didn't want to obviously. But I just knew that it was a totally necessary part of the whole process towards me getting well again. I explained that there was a meeting with my daughter way back in 2006. I felt quite confident that we were going to have a productive relationship once again, this was not to be the case, unfortunately. After our afternoon out together, we would send each other an occasional text and things seemed to me anyway to be going quite well. One day, though my illusions were totally shattered, I received a text message from her saying that she didn't want any further contact. I was dumbstruck, I couldn't believe it and I didn't want to believe it either!

The whole experience had left me completely devastated; it felt that my heart had been ripped from my chest. I was also finding this very tough to talk about, I remarked to Isobel. I kept thinking, had I done something wrong? I just didn't know and it was very confusing all round, to be honest. I needed to give Isobel the rundown of our relationship, pre-divorce that is. I had featured very heavily in my daughter's life. I used to

71

take her to swimming club three to five times a week, we would go out for walks, all the normal activities that families enjoy. My problem was that this situation was to change completely overnight and I just couldn't deal with it whatsoever. I did mention that Sian did offer up one of her pearls of wisdom at the time by stating to me that perhaps she's not ready to have a relationship with me just yet, I think she was probably spot on, after all, my daughter was at a difficult age at the time, roughly about sixteen and we all know about hormonal teenagers and all the stuff that goes with that! Having had a good think about what Sian had said hadn't made me feel any better, but it made me perhaps realise why she wanted to cut contact with me at that time in her life.

"What happened last summer 2017?" Isobel asked. Before we started any session, Isobel and I would have a little chat. I'd mentioned that my above situation had, in fact, changed slightly and I wanted to talk about it during our session.

"Well," I explained, "it was a blisteringly hot Sunday morning, so Sian and I decided to have a little drive out. The Cotswolds is very close by, so we thought we'd visit Broadway. Neither of us had actually been there before and so we chose to head off to the countryside on that momentous day. As we finished parking up, Sian went in her handbag to find her purse. My phone is always in her bag when we go out as I can't be bothered to carry it. She noticed a message light flashing away and just had a quick look at the screen. Her next words were 'you've got a message from your daughter.' I was totally taken aback, 'you're fucking joking me!' but she was right, it was from my daughter. I was so shocked. I hadn't had any contact for the best part of eleven years and although I was feeling elated, it was all a bit surreal, if I'm honest.

Isobel said, "WOW! How are things now between you and your daughter?" I explained that I was being very cautious about the whole situation because of what happened before, I couldn't allow myself to count my chickens. However, I did have reasons to hope that there would be a more successful outcome this time. She had for the first time passed onto me her phone number and home address, so this was making me feel a little bit more confident that things were moving in the right direction. I told Isobel that back in February 2018, we even shared a phone call! The call went okay and the only sour note was when she informed me that her older daughter was experiencing problems at school, in fact, the troubles were so bad that she was in the process of moving her to a new school. This traumatic experience that my daughter was currently suffering, immediately brought back to me all the bullying problems she'd also endured at her primary school, the end result being the same. I had to relocate her to a new school, where thankfully her situation worked out for the better. Further proof, if it were needed, is the fact that I regularly receive photographs of my two granddaughters, this is something I really appreciate, I told Isobel. For the first time I've been able to send birthday cards, Christmas presents etc., perhaps there really is light at the end of the tunnel.

"What's the current situation regarding your son, Phil?" I let out a huge sigh at the thought of trying to answer that difficult question. There is no hope at present, no hope whatsoever. I haven't seen or had any sort of contact with him in sixteen years! He was only eight when his mum and I split up, so maybe he's been influenced by his mother. I don't know for sure, but I've got my suspicions. My relationship with him was much the same as I'd had with my daughter; we did everything together. I took him to his first football match when he was just four years of age, this would happen very regularly over the next four years. When he started playing football for the under 7s, I was always there cheering him on and would also take him to the training every week. On one of his birthdays, he was even a matchday mascot at Brentford. We were very close at the time and I often wonder if he ever remembers any of this, I told Isobel. My love for my son and daughter can't be measured, I absolutely adore the pair of them, always have, always will and it still hurts me every day that I don't get to physically see them. To finish off my answer to Isobel's question, I said the only information I had regarding my son was that I'd heard that he was studying English Literature at Cardiff University of all places! This had made me incredibly proud indeed and I did wonder where he'd got his brains from!

To finish, I concluded that it was the result of the acrimonious break-up of the marriage and the stark fact that there was no contact between myself and my son and daughter that was almost certainly the reason that I eventually succumbed to my 'meltdown'. "It was all so bloody needless and served no good to anybody. Too much water has passed under the bridge now and I don't want to start slinging mud, there's just no point, but it doesn't stop me feeling angry about it, even now," I said. "Can we move on now, please? I'm starting to feel exhausted!"

The subject of bullying was about to rear its ugly head once more as we reached the end of session three. I explained to my lovely counsellor that I'd also been the victim of bullying in the workplace. I'd worked at the same company for the best part of twenty years and it was explained that the bullying was not just reserved for me. My boss at the time used his position of manager to generally make your life as difficult as he could. This would involve lots of mind games, threats would be made if you didn't work enough overtime and he would dock your bonus accordingly. The end result just generated a product of fear amongst the workforce and made it a very unhappy place to work at day in day out. For me personally, because I'd suffered bullying previously, it had probably made me a lot more sensitive to all that my manager would throw at me. I was never a wallflower and have always found it hard not to get involved when I see somebody being 'wronged'. So consequently, I would find myself in trouble with my boss on a regular basis. I told Isobel that at the time of the above problems, I was in my very early 20s, young and perhaps naive. And I also possessed a very fiery temper back then, so looking back now, it's easy to realise that there were certainly times I should have kept my 'big gob' shut. But at the time, I found it nigh on impossible to stand idly by while my old boss was 'dishing out his shit'.

Isobel was interested to see just how bad workplace bullying had affected me. I said that it had left a negative and lasting scar on my person. My tormentor was instigating his daily grief at a time that was not particularly long after the bullying at school, so it impacted on me very badly. "I'm so sorry to hear that, Phil, why do you think he chose to behave that way?"

I paused for thought, "Maybe he had his own issues? I don't know for sure. All I can say is that I've chosen to forgive him for his actions, it was a long time ago now and I'm not one to hold grudges." I finished by saying that eventually, it all ended badly for him as the company relieved him of his services. It became a great place to work for, the atmosphere completely changed for the better overnight and what's more, we ended up with a fantastic new boss.

My first three sessions had wiped me out emotionally; I was totally shot and I was left feeling like a complete physical wreck. I have to stress that over the course of the three sessions, it had been the hardest set of conversations, the outpouring of my soul that I'd ever undertaken in my whole life. I had put so much of myself into the whole counselling process, I had to, there really was no choice in the matter. Thankfully, there was a break of two weeks until my next appointment at Bradford House. It was two weeks that were desperately required at the time. I was shattered, but I felt very proud of myself. I'd been to emotional hell and back and I was still standing!

Session 4

My fourth session on the 21 February 2018 turned out to be a lot less troubling on my then very fragile mind. "Hello, Phil, it's very good to see you once again" I was now sitting opposite Isobel once more, ready to let my emotions pour out of me. I informed her in great detail everything that I'd experienced over the last fortnight. How 'fucked' I'd been, how it took over a week to feel anything like 'normal' again. And even when taking everything into account, I did actually feel a lot of personal pride and satisfaction at the way I'd dealt with my demons.

The topic of discussion to start that week was to be the subject of anger. My anger issues had plagued me all of my life. I'm certain this stemmed from my repressed emotional feelings concerning sexual abuse and the schoolyard bullying. This would explain my 'lashing out' at people, I said, perhaps it was my juvenile way of dealing with any situation I wasn't comfortable with, I don't know. The only thought I can be sure of is when I would end up in a scrap or something similar, I always felt like my 'pressure valve' had been released. I always felt better afterwards in a strange kind of way. A lot of hard work has been put in by myself over the years as I've matured and got older to work through my anger issues. It hasn't been easy, but I no longer 'lash out' and I am able to control my emotions in a much more constructive manner. I felt that for the time being at least, we should move on from my anger problems. It was almost certain in my mind that at some time in the future, we'd need to revisit the anger monster. I knew at some point the fallout would present itself to me. I say this because I'd had an emotional reaction quite quickly after my first few sessions. But I had a notion that this affliction was buried a lot deeper and that it might take a lot longer for my 'anger demon' to leave my head.

Next up, 'my lack of confidence'. For as long as I could remember, I'd had a confidence problem. "What do you mean, Phil?"

"The path of least resistance is the path I've always taken," I replied. A lot of thought and effort has happened on my part, I've tried to work out why this is so, but I always end up back at the beginning again and it frustrates the life out of me. People who know me might find it quite strange that I suffer from this particular problem because whenever I undertake any task, I do it to the best of my ability. It has to be stated at this point that I'm somewhat of a perfectionist; if I do a job, I do it properly, there's simply no other way in my book. The flipside to all this though, I explained, is that my need for any task to be done perfectly actually masks my pitfalls and insecurity. It explains why I've always tended to operate within my 'comfort zone'. This is especially prevalent concerning my working life, 'dead-end jobs' best describes my working career. Warehouse work and driving pretty much covers it!

"But those are honourable occupations," Isobel remarked.

"I know that really," I said, "but deep down, I know things could and should have been much better for me." I went further, "I'm certain that my lack of self-belief is connected to my past traumatic events and this has held me back, stopped me from really pushing myself."

"Perhaps you're being a bit hard on yourself, Phil?" It did sound like I was 'dissing' my jobs but my perceived high standards and all that! I started to tell Isobel all about my working career, how I'd left school in May 1982 and had found myself working in an airfreight company at Heathrow exactly one week later. Six/seven months were spent there and then I 'temped' for a short time. It was while I was temping that I began working at the company I'd spend the best part of twenty years at! The position worked out well for me there, I started as a temp and ended up as a supervisor. My role meant being in charge of all the deliveries that we received from France, Germany and the Far East!

"That sounds very impressive, Phil, you did really well." Deep down I knew she was right, but I wasn't totally convinced. I finished by telling Isobel that when I moved to

Swindon, I had to give the job up, the daily commute was just too much. This was when the next chapter of my working career started, I became a self-employed courier driver. I enjoyed this job; it was great being out and about. But as I've previously explained, all the very long mileage that had to be done was starting to get the better of me, along with the fact that the industry was no longer as lucrative as it once was. I did this for almost ten years and I really wasn't sure what I was going to do next. A mutual friend of ours worked part-time as a cabbie and he suggested that I should give it a go. This I undertook, although I did have my reservations about some aspects of the job, pissed passengers etc.! I continued to work on the cabs until the time of my 'meltdown'.

A large sip of water from my glass was required and then there was a slightly awkward silence for a few seconds. "I'll tell ya what it always feels like to me, Isobel. It feels as if I've got an angel on one shoulder and a demon on the other. They would constantly be shouting in both my ears, one trying to out-do the other. The angel would tell me that I could do anything that I put my mind to, the demon, on the other hand, would just tell me what a useless bastard I was!" This had always been the way of things. I knew that I'd wasted my education and had probably deserved all that was to transpire in my working life and it still pisses me off. However, I did say to Isobel that the demon on my shoulder may have won the battle when it came to my past self-belief and that he'd stopped me from pushing myself onto greater things. But I wasn't prepared to let the little demon fucker that was still in my head win the war, a war I'm absolutely determined to win and the eventual return of my good mental health.

We said our goodbyes and I left that lovely Victorian house knowing that the next session was going to be tough, really tough! We would be discussing my suicide attempts and as I walked down Milton road, I had a sick feeling in the pit of my stomach. The thought of the ordeal was bad enough, never mind talking about it.

Session 5

I had a very tough week leading up to my next appointment on the 28 February 2018. I'd experienced quite a few mini episodes of trepidation regarding my suicide attempts and I felt that it was going to be very traumatic session indeed. Even to this day, I always feel ashamed that I was weak to ever think that this was the only answer to my problems. To compound this issue further, I'd always considered myself a strong and resilient person but depression pays no respect to this whatsoever. At the time of my appointment, my depressed addled mind was absolutely convinced that there had only been three attempts to cut short my life. But I was to find out later that that couldn't have been further from the truth. I'd applied for my full medical records but at the time of my appointment, I still wasn't in possession of these.

As I made my way from the car park and down Milton Road, I can honestly say that I just as easily could have turned back and made my way home again. I didn't want to go through the process of opening up to Isobel once again and even though I'd managed to succeed in doing this previously, that particular week, I didn't feel anything like strong enough. I stopped walking and took a few seconds to compose and summon up the strength that was going to be needed to get through that next fifty minutes.

I suddenly sensed the feeling of déjà vu as I rang the bell at Bradford House, my stomach was doing cartwheels and it felt exactly the same as it had done on that very first occasion. Isobel greeted me with her lovely warm smile and this helped put me at ease a little. "Come in, Phil, how are you?" I didn't even give her the courtesy of a reply, I just smiled, I'd managed to get myself so worked up over the past week, I just wasn't my normal self. As we made our way down the narrow corridor I'm always pleasantly reminded of my late nan and granddad's house in Windsor. That was also Victorian and had the same room layout as Bradford House, quite a strange coincidence really. We took our seats in that rather drab nondescript room, nondescript in appearance, but if only those walls could talk, I always thought to myself every time I entered that room. I still felt very nervous and deep down I was praying that the session timewise would flyby. This was going to be very heart wrenching for me but it had to be done, there was no going back now.

I started our session with the words, "I'd like to talk about my suicide attempts please, Isobel" Ten words, nine of them very innocent looking and one other of a more menacing kind hid from the surface of the public view, the full intense agony of my ongoing situation. My pain, all the negative thinking, my shame, the regrets I had and the general sense of hopelessness that encompassed my whole being were contained in those ten little words. Those ten words had defined as a person for so long and I was sick to the back teeth of it. I had to exorcise this black ectoplasm before it destroyed me once and for all!

"Why did you want to end your life Phil?" were Isobel's first words to me. The question had penetrated my brain but I took a short time to answer.

"I was hurt so much, on a level that you can't even begin to describe" I replied. I went on to say that at that time, it felt like I had no control of my life, particularly the complete absence of any kind of relationship with my then young son and daughter. That situation was eating me up inside every single day and I couldn't find any way of positively dealing with it, it was a horrendous situation for me and also Sian.

"Unfortunately, Sian has always been on the receiving end of my wicked illness, it's so unfair on her. It leaves me feeling incredibly guilty and cuts me in half whenever it crosses my mind." I pointed out to Isobel that it was indeed me that walked out on my marriage but it was never my intention to walk away from my kids. Perhaps I was being slightly naive expecting my relationship with my son and daughter to remain the same, but we'd had a really close bond and that was the way I wanted it to continue, Isobel was told. It was explained that the separation had been very fractious but it was not the way I wanted it to be. I didn't want the kids to suffer any more than pain than was necessary.

The problem was that my ex seemed intent on war. She would go out of the way to be as difficult as she could. I just didn't understand it. She wanted to control every aspect of the situation. One example of this was when weekend visitations were arranged, I could only see my kids if my own mother came along as a chaperone! I can't tell you how mad this made me at the time. I mean just what did she think I would do? Abduct my own two kids! This would never have happened, they were my whole world and would never dream of hurting them or putting them in any sort of danger, the bloody woman was completely mad!

Isobel could see that even now; I was getting angry over this point. "I can see how frustrating that must have made you feel"

"It was so bloody stupid and unnecessary," I countered, "she had always been slightly controlling but she took it to stratospheric levels during those strained times, sad, so sad," I sighed. I'd had enough of talking about my ex-wife, I didn't want to spend the rest of my session slagging her off, there was just no point, but I had to finish that segment of the story by telling Isobel that the relationship between me and my offspring finally broke down because of my illness. "I had to cancel at the last minute a prearranged visit. At the time I was suffering one of my episodes, so I was in no fit state to travel or see anybody for that matter. Unfortunately for me, my bitter ex made the absolute most of the situation, probably telling my kids that I wasn't bothered about them and I didn't care. When the truth was, I adored my son and daughter, she knew this fact only too well but chose to be vindictive instead that proved to be the end of all contact from that point onwards."

"You must have taken that really hard," Isobel said. It had crushed me, I was completely devastated, it felt as though my heart had been ripped out at the time. She had taken them away from me and I just felt lost and hopeless. I didn't want to comprehend a future without them and the hurt I was feeling was unbearable.

Sian was always there for me during that very traumatic time. She has always been brilliant at giving me her total love and support, but I was heartbroken, it had killed me and I was literally a broken man. It was from that very devastating point in my life that I started to slowly spiral out of control. It had started, the very long road to my eventual meltdown in October 2017 had commenced.

Isobel's next question was fully expected but nonetheless, it still managed to knock the wind out of my sails temporarily. "When was your first overdose. Phil?" I had to think hard for an answer but replied by saying that I thought it was about nine months after the breaking off of contact with my two kids.

Basically, I think I struggled through those nine months until the day I reached a breaking point. I was totally exhausted; it takes a lot of energy out of you when trying to function to some kind of normality, when all you feel like doing is crawling into some dark corner and disappearing from the whole world. Inside I was still dying and I just wanted the pain to end. Sian was doing her very best to keep me going, but I couldn't see any other way out of my painful situation. On the day in question, Sian was at college. She was doing her two-year access course to attain the grades needed to start her studies into nursing. I remember getting up on that fateful day thinking that I'd just had enough of it all. I took all my medication tablets (I'd just picked up my prescription) and God knows how many painkillers and took myself back up to bed. My intention, I told Isobel, was to go to sleep and hopefully never wake up again!

I had to take a sip of water; this was bloody hard! I explained that this did not have the desired effect. I woke up four or five hours later feeling like absolute crap. "I couldn't even get that right! This made me feel like a total failure." As a result of this episode I was to be put under the care of the mental health team, this would be where I would meet Margaret Corkeran for the very first time. This happened way back in October 2003 and it had ultimately been her that had referred me to SWADS in December 2017. Leading up to my implosion I had been drinking heavily. Alcohol was my crutch but it was causing me harm and was making my depression worse with every drink. When I finally had in my possession my medical records, I discovered that it took me four days to seek out help. I had an appointment with a GP who did blood pressure, temperature checks, etc. and a phone call to the hospital poisons unit was made. They were of the opinion that my system would be clear of toxins by that point and no hospital visit would be needed.

More water was required, my mouth was as dry as the Sahara Desert. "Are you okay to carry on?" Isobel enquired.

"Yeah, I think so."

"Can you remember your second attempt, Phil?" At the time of our session, I hadn't been 100% sure but again with the help of my records I can tell you the reader that it was on the 7 April 2004. Not good timing on my part as it was my stepdaughter's sixth birthday! I said to Isobel that the reasons for my second attempt were pretty much the same as before. 1. I couldn't see my kids. 2. I was finding it impossible to adjust to life without them in it and 3. I could see no end to my suffering. "If there had been the slightest semblance of hope of contact at that time, I probably wouldn't have tried to end it all, but there was no hope, no hope at all" My situation was being further compounded by my ex-wife. I was making voluntary financial payments to her but this wasn't enough, so she decided to contact the child support agency. She maintained that these payments were 'gifts' and not regular child maintenance. "To cut a long story short, I contested her accusations and I had to attend my local magistrate's court."

I gathered all my financial evidence that was possible, this included pulling all my bank statements, etc. In court, I was able to prove that regular payments were being made by myself and the case against me was immediately thrown out by the judge. He then blasted the representative of the CSA that was attending court for wasting their and everybody's time. I and Sian left that court building feeling like justice had been done. The outcome of the court case had been a positive one but the stress of it all had taken its toll on us. The weeks leading up to our day in court had proved very worrying and traumatic indeed. "But it was an unnecessary and spiteful thing for my ex-wife to put us through," I exclaimed.

The second suicide attempt saw me end up in the hospital in the A&E ward. This would be the first time that I would have my stomach pumped. Copious amounts of various tablets had orally been taken again by myself. I stated to Isobel that I was quite sure that this occasion had been 'a cry for help'. I had been very desperate and frustrated at the situation I found myself in and the sheer hopelessness of my predicament had got the better of me. Once again, I was referred to the mental health team (for all the good it was doing for me at the time!) I had to apologise to Isobel because I really couldn't remember the date of my third attempt. My depressed foggy mind had put paid to that particular traumatic event. My medical records tell me now that it occurred on the 29 August 2005. Sixteen months had passed between episodes two and three, sixteen months of constant toil on my mind and soul had obviously taken its toll. 'The emotional dam' had to break at some point, there's only so much you can take until the waters break.

Horrifying details concerning my third attempt literally jumped off the page of my records. I'd 'ramped up' the amount of tablets and alcohol I'd consumed. I had arrived at A&E again, this time by ambulance. My stomach had to be pumped again! (not a nice experience I can tell you). Over thirty plus paracetamol tablets, forty-plus medication pills, lots of beer and a bottle of wine were downed apparently. A member of the nursing team told me that I was lucky to get to the hospital when I did and that an overnight stay on the observation ward was required. I said to Isobel that my suicide attempts had nearly crushed our relationship and lesser committed couples would have fallen by the wayside. It's fair to say that the guilt I feel because of my actions just can't be measured. It continues to eat away at my being even now as I write but it no longer controls me. I always pay it very healthy respect because it's a powerful emotion and I always try to remember all the grief that all of the above has inflicted upon Sian in particular.

That woman deserves a medal for valour!
She's been so strong for both of us!

"Quite how we survived that period of two years, I'll never know, Isobel, it was a miracle, really." Isobel looked just how I felt, completely shot! She glanced at the clock as did I, it was the end of what was a very punishing session. I felt absolutely fucked, devoid of any energy levels, wasted almost. I peeled my withered body out of the chair, that chair I'd sat on and spewed out my soul, it had been tough, but I knew only too well that there would be a lot more to come in the near future and it wasn't a very appetising prospect. But for now, I was just relieved to be saying my goodbyes to Isobel and I just hoped that I would make it home in one piece.

Chapter Fourteen

A Plum Is Not a Fruit!

The following true account you're about to read is from my point of view, slightly embarrassing. I felt the story was worth adding to my book for a couple of reasons. One it is, I feel, a welcome break from the very 'heavy subject matter' of the book and two, it still makes people piss themselves with laughter every time the account is wheeled out over a beer or two.

Towards the middle of January 2006, I started to experience problems around my 'one-eyed cat!' (my arse). I had been here before the 'nobbies' had afflicted me several times over the years and I thought that this was just another episode of the bloody thing! Generally, the symptoms would last one or two weeks, this would involve lots of uncomfortable sitting down and not wanting to go to the loo. Without going into too much graphic detail, going for a number two would be a case of excruciating agony, bog roll and arse coming together like friend and foe! Pain in the arse couldn't have been a more apt expression. At that time, I was working as a courier and obviously, this involved sitting down for long periods of time. As you can well imagine, after several hours of driving, my backside would be as itchy as a flea-ridden stray dog, not a very nice experience at all. Other people driving behind my van probably at times wondered what the hell was going on, the van would be going from side to side as I would shuffle in my seat in an attempt to scratch my neither regions.

However, this attack of the 'farmers' was beginning to turn into something completely different from previous episodes. It was a lot more painful and there was bleeding involved. This was giving me great cause for concern. On top of all this was the fact that my 'little appendage friend' was not very little at all, it felt like a very large grape! I decided that a visit to the doctor was required as the condition was getting worse and not better. An appointment was secured for the 2 February 2006 and to add to my woes, my consultation was to be with a female GP. This wouldn't be a problem for me at any other time, but this situation had the potential to get very embarrassing indeed. However, by the time of my appointment, I could no longer sit down to drive, the pain and general itching had made the task impossible and so consequently I couldn't work.

I reached the waiting room at my local GP surgery. I must have looked a right old sight as I tentatively lowered myself onto the uncomfortable plastic chair. Thankfully for me, my wait was very short and I made the walk to my allocated room, all the time trying to make it look like I hadn't shit my pants! I knocked on the door of the examination room, "Come in, please," said the voice coming through the door. Again, the parking of my arse was to be a slow and laborious task.

"Hello, Mr Green, what can I help you with?" A very frank and full account of my problem was told to my good lady doctor. "Okay, I'd better take a look, if you could take off your jeans, lower your underwear, climb up onto the treatment table and lie on your side please."

Oh blimey, I hadn't ever been asked to do that in a public area before, I thought as I had a good chuckle to myself. I'd even got to the point where I was actually no longer embarrassed by my predicament, a diagnosis was needed and quick. I was just so fed up with all the pain and itching and couldn't simply bear my situation any longer. The doctor began her examination around my back passage and out of the awkward silence came the words, "Oh my word! That's the largest thrombosed haemorrhoid I've ever come across."

"Thanks for that," I replied.

"That must be so sore," exclaimed my lady doc. Talk about a statement of the bleeding obvious I thought, but the word 'sore' really didn't cut it, the pain was horrendous.

I was told that a visit to A&E was urgently needed and I had to go straight away. "Bloody hell! Is it that bad?" I said.

"Yes, you've got an extremely swollen haemorrhoid and it needs urgent attention, I'll give the hospital a call right now." A feeling of relief and anxiety swept over me at that point; relief for very obvious reasons, but the anxiety bit kicked in when I started to think and wonder how they were going to deal with 'my plum' and just how painful was my ordeal going to be?

As I shuffled out of the surgery, I made a call to Sian. At that point in time, she was in the process of finishing her nursing degree and so would be at home. Studying along with her on that day was her friend Lina. She was hoping to work in the same profession and the two of them would very often study together. I filled Sian in with all the details, she picked me up and we raced off to the hospital. Lina decided to come too (perhaps she was bored of studying, I don't for sure) but they dropped me at the A&E entrance and off they went to find a parking space somewhere.

I got myself booked in at A&E and before I even had the chance to carefully park my very painful arse down, Sian and Lina walked in. We found some spare seats and got ourselves prepared for the potentially long wait. So, there we were. We sat on very uncomfortable chairs and hoping upon hope that my name would soon be called out. Time always seems to stand still in that 'department of doom and gloom'. You can actually feel all the pain and suffering that has ever occurred in that medical building and it always leaves me feeling like I should 'abandon all hope' (or is that just me!) With just a coffee and sweets vending machine along with bug-infested magazines to keep you company (why are they allowed in the hospital?) time just passes with interminable torture and would test the patience of a saint.

It wasn't long before I was dancing in my seat, the pain was getting increasingly worse, I didn't know what to do with myself. Walking was even more painful if that was possible and eventually, I had to ask for some much-needed pain relief. By that point, my throbbing unwanted friend must have looked like a flashing red stoplight. I reckoned if I'd dropped my cacks next to the roadside and pointed my arse at any oncoming cars, they would have stopped immediately!

Eventually, a poor overworked nurse appeared and called my name, Oh the relief! A&E was very busy as per normal, nurses were running around like headless chickens, they definitely deserve more pay! My cubicle wasn't quite ready for some reason, so we had to wait outside those 'soundproof curtains'. It was at this point that the day took another strange turn. Whilst Sian, Lina and I stood there waiting like spare wotsits at a wedding, the late Keith Chegwin popped his head around the corner of the department and said, "Oops, I think I'm lost!" His head disappeared back around the wall as quickly as it had appeared! All three of us looked at each other, perhaps not believing what we'd just seen. After our very short celebrity encounter, I was ushered into my allocated cubicle. It was now that I was to discover that I was going to be examined by a second female medic (no, I haven't got a problem with this!) But this was becoming more and more embarrassing for me and I was starting to get pissed off with the whole situation.

Once more I found myself on the examination table minus my cacks and lying prone on one side (this was starting to feel a bit kinky or is that just my dirty mind working again?) The next scene that was to play out can only be described as a comedy moment from a very famous set of comedy films from the 1960s/70s. Upon examining my rear end, my female medic literally shouted out, "Bloody hell! That's gotta be one of the biggest I've ever seen!" Now it has to be explained that although the department was busy, it was also pretty quiet. Her immortal words carried across that building as if they had been called out by the local town crier! Cue uncontrollable laughing and sniggering from the adjoining cubicles. Sian and Lina were literally pissing themselves. The line had been delivered at the perfect time and even I thought it was bloody hilarious. It was so, just so funny, it could have been another funny scene from one of the aforementioned set of films and it felt like I was the 'butt' (pardon the pun) of everybody's joke, but you can't beat a bit of innuendo I say!

The lady doc carried on her examination of my 'plum'. She then explained that my unusual case may be of interest to some junior docs that were shadowing on the ward. "Would you mind if they came and took a look, Phil?" Well, I didn't even get a chance to answer her question, she hurried off leaving me open-mouthed. At this point in proceedings, Sian decided to poke her head through the curtains.

"Let's have a look then," she said. All the time a huge grin was plastered across her face.

"Piss off," was my reply, I wasn't too keen for her to further examine my 'ring'. After all, there was more of that to come from the junior docs at any moment.

"Where's she gone now?" Sian enquired.

"She wants to showcase my arsehole," came my reply, more laughter from Sian and Lina was to follow, they were having a great laugh at my expense.

I was beginning to feel like some Victorian circus freak and before long, my medic returned with half a dozen or so junior colleagues in tow, all eager, no doubt, to inspect my newfound friend. I was asked again if it was okay for me if these young medical students could take a look at my enlarged appendage. This time I was given an opportunity to answer. I really had gone past the point of caring too much, I mean how much more dignity could I lose?

"Yeah, knock yourselves out," came my reply. The junior docs took it in turn to study my thrombosed haemorrhoid. They all seemed to have the same bemused look upon their faces and I could tell by the thinly veiled comments and occasional sniggers that my predicament was a truly unique and interesting case. One or two of them were braver than the rest. They needed a much closer look and from my perspective were a little too close for my comfort. In their minds, I must have had some sort of alien life form attached to my backside and were just waiting for a razor jawed monster to burst out of the top of my swollen plum! I imagined them telling people years later of the time that they were in training and had come across this poor individual with a rather unusual case of piles and perhaps my condition would even become a topic of conversation at a dinner party.

After probably about five minutes (although it seemed a lot longer) my ordeal was over. The young doctors all thanked me for allowing them an inspection of my bum. I was just glad it was over, to be honest. My lady doc went off to see if there was a surgeon available to carry out what she described as a 'minor procedure'. *Minor procedure!* I thought, *Bloody hell! it wasn't anything of the sort in my head.* All sorts of horrible images were flashing across my mind, just how were they going to deal with my heavily swollen plum? Thankfully, my wait was very short. The surgeon walked in and along with what felt like the world and his wife began to examine my backside.

"My word! You're a big fella aren't you," exclaimed the very polite surgeon.

Oh great! I thought to myself. This can't be very good but he managed to reassure me that although the haemorrhoid was big, it wouldn't present a problem. I felt some relief hearing his words, but I'd be lying if I said I wasn't worried at potentially what was to come.

"We will carry out the procedure right away, I just need to find an assistant to help me."

"What here, right now?" I nervously replied.

"Yes, I'll be back in a few minutes." Those few minutes seemed like an hour, I was literally crapping myself, but I also wanted it sorted. The pain was by now excruciating, to say the least. My surgeon returned with a colleague; these were the two men that were being tasked to go to war with my unwanted swelling.

"Okay, Mr Green, my assistant is going to put a small injection on both sides of your groin."

"What the fuck."

"Oh don't worry too much, it will only sting a little and afterwards you won't feel a thing," said the assistant. This didn't convince me at the time but he turned out to be right. As you can imagine, my heart was jumping out of my chest at this point, I was not looking forward to this at all. The first injection goes in, the stinging was no less painful than I was already experiencing. (*Shit! that bloody hurt*, I thought.) The second equally painful injection goes in and before very long, the pain I'd been suffering for so long was beginning to subside. The surgeon approached my nether regions and with some slight pulling and tugging about and apparently some tying off, which felt like he was tying a pair of shoelaces, the blood supply to the haemorrhoid was eventually cut off. The job was done. He explained that the haemorrhoid would go necrotic and fall off into my underwear (that's nice I thought).

The procedure had seemed so simple (as if it was no more difficult than tying up a knot in a piece of string). But as far as I was concerned, I was just so happy and relieved that my problem was no more. I couldn't thank the two gentlemen enough. It had been a very painful ordeal and a feeling of immense relief swept over me. I still hobbled out of that A&E

department but it was much more pain-free than the walk into that building, I can safely assure you!

Chapter Fifteen
The Dog Takes a Nip!

It's Tuesday night, Sian is watching one of those cookery programs that I pretend to hate, England is playing Italy but I've not much interest in friendlies and up until very recently, watching England is very often a painful experience. I can tell you that Sian is feeling under par, which is noticeable as she has always been the more upbeat of the two of us and I'm pretty good at reading people, Sian in particular. I ask if she's okay and replies that she is feeling a bit crappy but is okay and not to worry. This doesn't reassure me and I immediately get this horrible feeling in the pit of my stomach, which I always liken to a washing machine, my guts tumbling around on as fast spin.

Sadly, my loyal demon wakes from his slumber after not showing himself for a couple of months. I haven't missed him one little bit and I suddenly realise and ask, "Where the fuck have you been? Am I bloody crazy? Why am I asking him his whereabouts? You stupid sod!" I start to get this familiar feeling in my head. It's hard to describe but I see and feel it as black fog.

The cookery programme finishes and Sian is obviously exhausted as a result of working long shifts and extra shifts to cover my sorry arse. The guilt is kicking in again even following assurances that I am under no pressure in any shape or form. Try telling that to my little friend in my head though! He never listens to reason as his mission is to screw me up and spit me out. Sian loves her bed, but I know that as she climbs the stairs this time, it's out of necessity and not happy pleasure.

For some reason, I switch channels and watch the remaining minutes of the England game. To my surprise, they're only bloody winning! Perhaps England's manager is beginning to get these overpaid prima donnas playing at long last. But no, this is England we are talking about here. We gave away an ever so slightly dodgy penalty given with thanks by VAR. Our friendly German referee pointed to the spot and the goal was duly scored. Now, in normal circumstances with this game being a friendly, the result of the game which occurred in the 89th minute would not have bothered me in the least, but I was ruminating over how Sian was feeling, which compounded my sad mood more than usual. I took myself to bed but tossed and turned as my guilty mind was working overtime. The logical side of my head is literally fighting the little fucker with his negative attitude and I pray that he would stop. I can't find peace of mind, no matter how hard I try. The black fog is lingering, but I am aware that it doesn't feel nearly as thick as usual.

My mood has been much better in the past couple of months and had not had a visit from my demon. Maybe I've become stronger. Up until now, I have not won a battle with my little friend, but this time, I could feel an inner strength that I have not felt for years.

You are not going to win, I thought, *enough, I want to sleep now.*

I guess after a good hour, I dropped off to sleep. This is something I don't usually have trouble with as although I am feeling better, my illness leaves me constantly tired. I wake up again at 2:30 am, my mind is active and I found myself ruminating over negative thoughts for a short while, but I'm managing to fight them off and dismiss them quickly from my head and I fall back off to sleep. Bliss.

Rather surprisingly, I wake up feeling ok. I have a workout but don't push myself too hard as I'm mindful that I've moved away from the edge of the cliff and could easily trip over the edge. I walk to the shop and read the paper. No drama.

This shouldn't be taken the wrong way but Sian returned home from having her hair done and although I was obviously pleased to see her, those negative thoughts were forcing their way back into my head once again. Subconsciously, seeing Sian must have triggered these thoughts and try as I might to push them aside, Sian must have known there was something wrong. I quietly went to bed early and Sian tackled me in the morning. In the past, I would have brushed her off with the usual line of 'I'm fine' but I'm making a real effort to talk to her when I'm feeling rough. I explained how I was feeling and she gave me the assurance I needed. I spent the rest of the afternoon subdued until time for a weekly counselling session that evening.

Chapter Sixteen

Blues and Soul – Part 3

Sessions 6 and 7

My sixth session with Isobel, which was at the start of March 2018 was basically a 'review' of my previous appointments, an 'overview' of everything we'd discussed previously. Although I was starting to feel better, I explained that where I was, was by no means anywhere near my final destination. I went further to tell Isobel that 'yes' that probably for the first time I felt some hope regarding my future and maybe, just maybe, I could see the little white spot of light at the end of my torturous mental tunnel.

A three-week break followed session 6 and it was reassuring to meet up with my lovely counsellor once again. For some strange reason, I was actually missing my unremarkable little room at the back of Bradford House, perhaps it had become my little comfort blanket. That room should really have felt like the last place I'd want to drag myself off to but I think at that very troubling time, it became my 'emotional crutch'. Perverted as it might seem, I think I was finding the whole process of unloading all my emotional crap very addictive in a weird sick kind of way. I've previously alluded to the fact that my earlier sessions had hit me really hard physically and emotionally but offloading all the years of hurt that I'd carried on my person, the unshackling of the heavy chains of my depressive illness seemed to give me a 'high'. That is sick, isn't it? How could discussing distressing subjects such as child abuse and bullying leave me feeling good? I can only come to the conclusion that the spewing out of my soul was actually doing me a lot of good, perhaps more than I realised and the only thing I was sure of at the time was that I needed my next fix!

The topic of discussion for session 7 was to be on the subject of my old foe 'guilt' and especially how it related in my mind regarding Sian. It cannot be understated just how much my fucking horrible illness has afflicted Sian over the course of our almost 17 years together. She has withstood the constant onslaught that my illness has thrown at her and still, she stands strong (I really don't know how). She has sucked up all of my suicide attempts and all the emotional worry that goes with that. The numerous other depression episodes that have eaten away at her very being and I make no bones about it when I say that it is her that has kept me going throughout all of my mental troubles. It's her I can never say thank you enough to and perhaps now you can begin to imagine as to why I feel as guilty as I do.

"Sian is constantly tired," I exclaimed to Isobel, "and it's all down to me. No human being should be made to go through all that she has, it's just not fair, not fair at all."

"It isn't your fault, Phil, it's your illness after all," countered Isobel. I knew that, of course, but my depressed foggy head can't comprehend that simple fact, it never does!

"The guilt is my problem, Isobel, it's my responsibility, illness or not and it doesn't feel good knowing that it's my actions that are badly affecting Sian." At the time of this session, Sian was having a wobble. She really was having a tough time of things and trying to hold the family together was proving very difficult. To an outsider, this stark fact would be hardly surprising given the whole situation that she found herself in, lesser mortals would have fled the scene or it would have finished them off altogether, one or the other! I repeated again to Isobel that I was starting to improve, but as far as Sian's situation was concerned, the horse had already bolted! It was too late to slam the stable door shut, the damage to Sian had already been inflicted.

Most of our appointment was taken up on the above subject. The session had proved once again very taxing. I was wiped out; my eyes were very sore. Just how much more could my mind and body take? I didn't know, but I had to carry on with the fight. The session was ended with the revelation that I had decided to write a book. "Really," Isobel exclaimed,

"Yeah, I'm going to write an account of my life journey, it will be all about my life living with depression, but it will be written in a way that I hope can also help other people suffering in similar circumstances." Isobel was taken aback somewhat by my piece of news, she gave me a strange look, perhaps wondering if she'd heard me right.

Eventually, she said, "That's brilliant, Phil, fantastic news." Considering just how bad my illness had been affecting me at our first get together and to a large extent still was. It really was no surprise that anybody at that stage could have thought I'd been capable of stringing more than two words together, never mind trying to write a whole book!

Sessions 8, 9 and 10

My next three appointments during April 2018 were for me personally a lot less traumatic, in as much there were to be no real heavy subjects discussed between myself and Isobel. This was down to the fact that we'd already ploughed our way through what I considered were the main triggers that had kickstarted my depression in the first place. That situation would change somewhat the following month when I was to receive my full medical records from my GP surgery. However, there was still plenty to discuss with Isobel.

I explained that the previous week had left me struggling to cope with my problems. This had come about because Sian had written a very heartfelt account of her personal experience of living with somebody that suffers from a long-term mental health issue. In a previous chapter of this book titled *'The Truth Hits the Heart'*, I described in detail how reading that personal account had completely poleaxed me and had left me feeling very guilty and traumatised at the same time.

Session 8 was spent going into great depth about all of my concerns. The guilt, the sadness and regrets that I'd felt when reading all that heart-crushing piece of writing that Sian had expertly put down on paper. I even hammered home the point to Isobel that what I'd read felt like she was talking about somebody else completely, not me! "That must have been a very difficult experience for you, Phil?" Isobel had delivered that line in what I considered to be a very understanding and compassionate manner. I think she knew just how I was feeling at that particular time. The thing was, it had hit home really hard, it was like a hard punch to the stomach, the wind had been knocked out of my sails that was for sure. I and Isobel had really picked out the bones during that session and I had gone some way to dealing with that particular demon, even if I hadn't totally beaten him at that point.

The following week soon arrived, session 9 beckoned. "How are you feeling, Phil?" Isobel enquired.

"I'm feeling really, really tired" came my reply. "I have a feeling that the whole counselling process has caught up with me, Isobel"

"That's hardly surprising, we've covered some pretty heavy subjects, some of those were very distressing for you, Phil" She was 100% correct. I'd found it extremely hard disclosing horrific and painful experiences during my time in that little back room in Bradford House and it had wiped me out.

"I've never had so many early nights. I have to drag my sorry bag of bones up to bed most evenings by nine o'clock." On a more positive note, I was starting to rationalise my thoughts better. Thinking things 'in a new way', although I say 'new' because I'm not entirely sure if the way I was thinking was new or not. It had been such a long time that I was able to think with anything like a clear head that it was impossible for me to remember to be quite honest. All I was sure of, though, was that my thought processes felt very different, it was easier for me to take things in and make decisions. If I didn't know better, it was almost as if some surgeon had given me a new head! "We can only wait and see if my new way of thinking is something I've learned or perhaps the old Phil is starting to re-emerge, 'only time will tell'," I stated.

I returned to the subject of tiredness. "The extreme fatigue I'm feeling is probably the result of years and years of bottling up my emotions, they have been allowed to fester and they've got stronger and stronger with each passing year". My mouth was very dry, I took a sip of water and then I went further. "My incarcerated emotions had literally got stronger than me, it had happened right under my nose and there was absolutely nothing I could do to stop it." Isobel asked me if I was okay to carry on?

"Yeah, sure, I'm ok." It has to be explained that the power of the illness that is depression will knock over and flatten the strongest of people. I was and still am a very strong person. It's how I managed to function and carry on for over four decades and although I tried as hard as I did, it eventually took me down with no mercy shown. I described to Isobel that my situation at that time felt as if 'my emotional dam had given way, the pressure had proved too much and instead of water rushing through my cracks, a steady flow of black demon juice was seeping out of my pores'. I say seeping because my counselling was never going to be an overnight fix. It was going to take some considerable time for my emotional shit to finally leave my system. Nonetheless, the colonic demon irrigation had started and even if I was feeling completely washed up, I knew deep down that with all the hard work and effort I was putting in on a daily basis, the war was slowly being won.

A two-week break followed due to our trip to Cornwall. Session 10 turned out to be of a very light nature. We spoke about my 'small bumps in the road' that I'd experienced in the weeks leading up to the Cornwall trip. These so-called small hiccups were fully expected on my part. They were a necessary part of the whole getting better process as far as I was concerned. This pragmatic thinking was a positive sign in my eyes, the fact that I could look at these small setbacks in a positive manner was real progress for me. It has to be stated that although this was all very good, I was still finding myself. These positive thoughts were slightly alien to me and I was still trying to come to terms with it all. I explained to my warm counsellor that the small bumps would have badly affected my mood in the past. My mind was on a negative default setting and there would have been occasions when I just couldn't have dealt with the problem constructively and a depressive episode would more than likely have occurred afterwards.

Next to guilt, my biggest demon foe was rumination. Guilt was the result of my depression, but it was my ruminating that had contributed so much negative ammunition towards my illness. There simply is no living being that could beat me up and inflict as much damage as I was able to do to myself. I was a world champion at the art of the heavy negative thinking, rumination was king. It had got so natural to me and most of the time I was totally unaware that I was doing it. However, and much to my surprise, I'm not allowing these damaging imposters to enter my mind. They're unable to sit in my head festering away, they have no hold or control on me any longer. It was not an issue that I thought could be tamed as easily as it has so far appeared. I've put a lot of hard work in, so perhaps the rewards are being reaped? I don't know for certain, but hey, I'll take that for now. Nothing will be taken for granted on my part, I will continue to be very vigilant. I know this ruminating demon too well and I will fight fire with fire if necessary, to make sure he never shows his ugly mug ever again!

Session 11 would follow in three weeks due to Isobel being away on holiday but before that would take place, I was to receive my full medical records. Whereupon I was to discover some rather disturbing long-forgotten facts that would prove very difficult for me to digest and deal with.

Session 11

The three-week break soon whizzed by and before I knew it, I found myself knocking on the front door of Bradford House once again. The date was the 16 May, not an important date specifically but it proved to be of some significance to me personally. It was the day that I was to receive my full medical records, it was also the same time that my preconceived memories regarding my previous suicide attempts were to be blown out of the water. During that auspicious day, I only had time to browse very quickly at my records but still, it proved long enough for me to discover the correct amount of times that I'd attempted to end my life.

Isobel greeted me at the door, she gave me a big smile, it was a smile that I was getting used to seeing and it always managed to put me at ease from the off. We chatted for a few minutes, I asked about her holiday, had she had a good time, general chit chat. I informed Isobel that my medical records had arrived and that I'd found some very distressing facts concerning my suicide attempts. "I'm absolutely shell shocked," I exclaimed.

"Why is that, Phil?"

"Well, I always thought that there were only three previous suicide attempts, but in actual fact, there were seven! How the hell could I have forgotten that not so little fact?" Isobel looked slightly shocked at my revelation.

"How does that make you feel?"

"Bloody rotten! I repeat how the fuck could I have totally forgotten the extra four occasions when I had tried to end it all?" To anybody that's never suffered a mental illness, this fact probably seems absolutely inconceivable, I mean, just how is it possible? The answer to it is really quite simple. Depression robs you of your memory, it erases certain traumatic events from your mind, maybe it's a safety net. Who knows for sure? However, I can honestly state that this has certainly happened to me, it's hardly surprising in my case when you think about it. I mean carrying around all of my shit for over forty years has almost certainly contributed to my loss of memory. I have no doubts about that.

"That must have come as a massive shock to you, Phil, reading all about those facts in black and white?" The truth was that I felt completely devastated but what was also troubling me was the fact that these very troubling events had only made themselves known to me earlier that day. My head hadn't had the required time to take it all in and process it in a constructive manner. This had the potential to blow up in my head at a later time and so consequently, it was causing me no end of worry.

I explained to Isobel that discovering the very traumatic information had ended with me receiving another 'blow' to my brain. "I feel like a punch-drunk boxer, that's just exactly how I feel at the moment. Perhaps this 'hit' and all the other hits I've taken over the years have added to memory woes."

The guilt monster had started to give me a kick. I felt it building up during the session. The kick to my shins was reminding me of all the hurt I'd inflicted on Sian and it didn't make me feel very good. A physical symptom had started up too, the tumble dryer in my stomach was warming up, spinning slowly but it was working itself up for a full spin at any moment. (*Fuck, here we go again,* I thought to myself.)

I finished the water in my glass, God this was hard. I hadn't expected this at all, in my mind we'd already covered what I considered were the most horrifying details of my past but here we were again. But this time my head was dealing with traumatic events that I wasn't prepared for in any shape or form. Isobel suggested that I should try and go easy on myself in case it had a detrimental effect on my recovery. She had made a very good point. I was making good progress and I was absolutely determined that that was not going to happen. But events had shaken me to the core and I'd been knocked off my feet. I was also very worried about what might happen next. "I think I may well struggle over the next few days. This isn't going to be easy for me but I will sleep on it, try and take it for what it is and not allow myself to ruminate if at all possible," I told Isobel.

The session had flown by once again, it had been a very tough appointment. The walk back to collect the car proved difficult. I was glad to be going home.

The dates of my four forgotten suicide attempts are as follows:

24 October 2005

Alcohol + 28 antidepressant pills, 60+ paracetamol pills + unknown amount of painkiller pills.

17 February 2006

Alcohol + unknown amount of antidepressant pills, 55/60 painkiller pills.

12 December 2008

65/70 paracetamol + unknown amount of antidepressant pills.

23 August 2013

The details are a bit sketchy regarding this episode. This date is our wedding anniversary, but we were experiencing some domestic problems around that time and Sian had decided to visit a friend and stay overnight. I decided to drink and take an unknown amount of antidepressant pills and painkillers knowing that she wouldn't be back in time to probably save me. Unfortunately for me, I'd failed again. Sian found me in bed asleep early the next morning. I woke up feeling very drowsy but very much alive! A trip to A&E was to quickly follow (God, I was literally sick to death of that place!)

As you can see, it doesn't make for good reading and I wonder to myself, *How the hell am I still here?*

Sessions 12, 13 and 14

My worst fears concerning the possible emotional fallout had proved to be correct. The following week was tough, very tough! I still couldn't comprehend the fact that somehow, I'd managed to completely forget 'four' suicide attempts. A great sense of shame had enveloped me, feeling like utter crap didn't cut it. I've felt bad plenty of times in my life but this was on another level. The whole situation during that week stank to high heaven. I kept asking myself in my head over and over again, "How could you have forgotten, you muppet!"

Eventually, Wednesday came back around and it was time for session 12. The trauma in my mind continued to remind me as I fully described to Isobel the events of the past week. I think I was still in a state of shock to be perfectly honest, trying to digest all of the terrible facts was proving impossible. My poor swede seemed unable or it was simply incapable of grasping the grizzly details, I just didn't want to know. However, although I was feeling absolutely rotten, the most positive aspect was the realisation that I seemed to be keeping my mental wellbeing in check. "This situation would without any doubt have taken me down in the past, Isobel, it would have been far too traumatic for me to handle."

"Well done, Phil, that's a very positive sign, you seem to be making progress," Isobel remarked. I was making good progress, albeit very slowly. I was more than happy to continue to take one day at a time, it was serving me well and I had no intention of sabotaging my recovery.

To the uninitiated, it might seem slightly strange to grasp the fact that at the age of fifty-two, I was starting to learn to 'think' again. Depression clouds your judgement. How you see and feel certain events are not necessarily the same as other people. You tend to have a very warped negative attitude and opinion to conversations and situations that are playing out before you. You convince yourself that what you're thinking is 100% correct but very often it's not the case at all. For so many years, my illness didn't allow me to 'see' this fact and it's only just recently that this has been possible due to my ability to think a lot clearer, thanks in part to my recovery.

Isobel wanted to know how Sian was bearing up. She knew I'd been very worried about her and my answer to her was that she was in fact, struggling badly. "For the last couple of months, Sian's not been good at all. I'm still very concerned for her; I just don't know what to do."

"I'm starting to feel better and I'm continuing to do all the correct things as regards to my recovery, but Sian has got no better whatsoever. I'm at a total loss, Isobel."

"That's got to be tough, Phil?" I paused for a short time; it was very upsetting for me. A sense of frustration was what I felt at that time, things were improving for me and I kept thinking that maybe there had been some sort of transference on my part. Had all my shit and constant problems leaked into Sian's system? It would be very plausible. She had sucked up all of my problems and been there for me. Was she now suffering a breakdown too?

"All I can do on my part is to continue to love and support her through this very tough time and hope that she comes out the other side sooner rather than later," I said to Isobel. Time waits for no man and before we knew it, the session had come to an end. I felt like I'd been put through the mangle once again. I know that my appointments with Isobel are doing me a lot of good and are, in fact, working for me but it was all getting a bit slightly wearing. Post-session found me walking down Milton road feeling as if I'd just had a lobotomy!

Session 13 followed at the end of May and I was beginning to feel like a lodger at Bradford House. Coming to terms with what I found in my medical records was starting to register with me. It hadn't been easy but it obviously needed time to sink in. I wasn't out of the woods just yet but nonetheless, progress was being made and that was all that mattered in the long run. Better still was the improvement in Sian's general wellbeing. She was a lot more bright and bubbly and the worst seemed to be behind her. This resulted in me feeling so much better too. She had been through a very turbulent time, which at times had left me sick with worry. It needs to be explained that at that particular point in time, I hadn't taken another look at my med records, as you can imagine it was something, I was very reluctant to do. However, it was a task that had to be undertaken, facts had to be pulled that pertained to this book and perhaps more importantly as far as I was concerned, I needed to gain peace of mind.

Isobel asked me how the writing was going. "Very well, although the subject matter I was currently writing was of a very heavy nature: the bullying, sexual abuse and my suicide attempts," I told her. "The process of putting it down on record has left its mark on me, it's been pretty tough that's for sure!"

"I'm looking forward to reading it," Isobel told me very enthusiastically.

"I would hope that people will want to read it, it is very heavy in parts but that's the subject I'm writing about. I've tried to make the book as interesting as possible by featuring accounts of happier times as well but it's not easy." One of the main reasons that I decided to write this book on the subject of depression was that it might prove helpful and informative for people that might be in a similar situation as myself. I mean, I'm just an ordinary guy off the street with what I think is a good story to tell but if the book can help people, then so much the better.

A drink of water was needed, my mouth felt like Gandhi's flip-flops! I glanced at the clock, we still had ten minutes to go. "It's funny," I said, "I always worry beforehand that I'm gonna turn up for a session and have nothing to say, I'm gonna 'run dry' and there will be long awkward silences," I say this because normally I'm not the world's greatest talker! Isobel gives me a rather puzzled look as if to say that she doesn't quite believe in the statement I've just made. (But it's true, ask anybody that really knows me.) Perhaps the reason the above has never happened is most probably down to the fact that during these sessions, I've been putting in 110% effort in my bid to get well again.

Another appointment came to a close, it would be two weeks before I saw Isobel again.

Session 14 arrived predictably quick, it was 13 June and once again I find my old bones sitting opposite Isobel. My very kind counsellor was informed that Sian had written her second contribution to my book. It's titled *'Hanging in There'*. "How did that make you feel, Phil?" I explained that although it did make for painful reading, it hadn't hit home quite as hard as the first account had done. As sure as night follows day though, my old nemesis 'guilt' resurfaced (what is it with this demon, can't he cut me some slack?) We discussed this very sore point in great detail as we'd done before. "This bastard demon just eats away at my very soul," I exclaimed, "He just won't leave me alone!"

At that stage I was finding the writing very difficult. I knew that it would be but it was also part of the whole process of me getting well again. The extreme tiredness was a big factor still, although it was not causing me any great concern. It was beginning to feel somewhat normal to me but nonetheless, it was very tough to deal with. Despite all of the above though, I was starting to positively believe that my personal war was starting to be won. I was able to keep my various demons in check, they were no longer ruling my mind in the damaging way that they'd managed previously. For maybe the first time, it was me kicking their arse and it felt bloody good!

Discussing my guilt had proved once again very taxing and Isobel gave me an understanding look. She knew I'd been through the wringer but somehow I felt confident that the fact that we'd now covered all of my major issues, that perhaps I can finally state that 'Phil Green was back in the room!'.

Chapter Seventeen

Cornwall Capers, Oh, and the Dog Is Still Trying to Take a Bite...

Just when I think I'm making good progress in my personal battle with this bleeding illness, I got a reminder that I've still got a very long way to go on this matter. Sian and I have just returned from a well-earned break from the lovely part of this country that is Cornwall. We both really enjoyed ourselves so much, it was great. Apart from our first day there, the weather decided to put its sun hat on, something I wished I'd done as I went on to burn my head! At the time of writing, my head is peeling like mad and it looks very unsightly indeed!

We decided that we'd spend our first day visiting the doc's home in Port Isaac aka 'Port Wenn'. The weather was far worse than expected, very grey and dull and with that horrible drizzly rain that just seems to stick to you. I had my shorts on, which is perfectly normal for me now that we were into April, but thankfully, I had the foresight to wear a fleece top as it was bloody cold! Sian being the more sensible out of the two of us was wearing jeans, so it was consequently taking the piss out of me! We did the obligatory tourist thing by taking snaps outside the various characters houses that appear in the show. But with the continuing drizzle raining down on us, a trip to the 'Doc's pub' to seek refuge and warmth was called for. Nothing beats a nice pint in front of a roaring hot fire and we enjoyed a very pleasant couple of hours sat in that famous pub.

After visiting Port Isaac, we drove to our hotel in Tintagel, perhaps not surprisingly to most people that know us, our venue was a pub! With a lovely big breakfast thrown in with the price of the room, we couldn't have been happier. It has to be said that the food was way above the standard we'd expected, it was very, very good. If you ever find yourselves wanting to visit the area, I can highly recommend the King Arthurs Arms, you won't be disappointed.

After breakfast, we walked the short distance to visit Tintagel Castle. We then decided to take a two-mile walk to a pretty bay called Trebarwith. There was also the prospect of a nice cold beer at the end of the walk. The pub in question had been recommended to us by one of the castle's members of staff. Now I use the term 'walk' very loosely here. Sian decided that we should take the coastal path and what with me being a 'townie', I was expecting some sort of well-worn stoned path. No, that was not the case at all and I feel I should explain at this point that Sian just loves an adventure. On some of these so-called 'walks', it has been known for us to find ourselves hiking through animal inhabited fields, which are very often known as 'National Trust Nature Trails'. These often resemble mud baths and I'm certainly no hiker!

On this occasion, I was enjoying the walk. Thankfully it wasn't too muddy, but it was interesting, to say the least. As I've already mentioned, this walk was taking place after our visit to the castle. Anybody who has visited this historic part of our country will attest that with all the very steep steps and inclines at the site, you will be left feeling like you've had a good workout. The castle saves the best till last. To exit the site, you have to walk up a very steep gradient that I would say is probably a 1/20 incline and must be at least a quarter of a mile in length. By the time we reached the top, my calf muscles were literally on fire. Looking across to Sian, I knew she felt the same pain!

The 'path' we were walking on was only about a foot wide and was a mixture of embedded stones and dried up mud. This made the process of walking in a straight line somewhat difficult and I was particularly worried that I might turn over my very weak right ankle. Something I'd done many times when I use to play football. Occasionally the path would get wider but it never lasted long and I could tell Sian was really enjoying her 'adventure'. Frequently, she would tell me to shut and stop moaning, but I tend to enjoy my walk more if I'm not worrying about where I'm going to plant my size 10s. I kept thinking to myself and wondering why that a path that perhaps millions of people had walked on over the years was so bloody small! Oh, here we go again I thought as we approached an upcoming stile that meant only one thing in my mind – animals and piles of shit! I felt strangely disappointed at the lack of animals that weren't there to greet us but there was still plenty of great steaming 'Richards' to avoid. Sian 'Captain Scott' was of course in her element but at least this 'expedition' was not as mud-filled and animal incident-packed as previous country jaunts.

The next hazard we had to negotiate was a very sharp bend right near the cliff edge. The weather was very warm, but the wind was blowing a very strong gale as we were right next to the sea. It was a miracle that we weren't blown off as we turned the corner, the strength of the wind was simply incredible. It made you realise just how small and insignificant you really are compared to the force of Mother Nature. It was hard to build up a head of steam on those ankle-turning paths, more stiles and lots of puddles were overcome until eventually, the bay of Trebarwith came into view. Sian kept telling me to just think about that nice cold pint of beer that would be waiting for me. She really didn't have to keep reminding me, Gandhi's flip flops and all that, my mouth was as dry as the Gobi Desert. We had the long climb down the cliff to negotiate and then we'd be there. Heaven!

A pint and a half of 'rattler' were duly ordered (a lovely local cider) and we sat ourselves down on an outside table that totally overlooked the bay. It was an amazing sight to behold. You could see why surfing is so popular down in Cornwall, the waves that were crashing in were huge and pretty impressive. As we enjoyed our drinks Sian suggested that we could walk back to Tintagel by way of the main road and this would be easier on my knackered old knees. The thing was though, I knew that Sian the adventurer didn't really want to do that and truth be told I wasn't too keen either. After all, we were on holiday and I felt that would go against the spirit of the 'adventure'. I said no to Sian, we will walk back the way we came. I think she was pleased that I'd said that, but as I looked up over the top of my pint and to the sight of the huge steep path back up the side of the cliff, I got a reminder from my already wiped out knees that they really didn't fancy it at all!

We walked down to the bay and purchased a couple of ice creams, sat on a rock and watched the tide come in. It had been a lovely visit, but now we had to summon up the energy for the walk back. The two-mile walk each way would not normally present a problem, we would very often walk double that and in half the time but this was no easy walk. It was full of potential hazards. You would've thought that we would have remembered most of them but that didn't stop me falling head over tit on one of the stiles, much to Sian's obvious amusement! The rest of the walk back passed by without any further incident to myself or Sian but we did have one small problem to overcome still. The walk we were on meant to get to the hotel. We had to walk up that massive hill I mentioned earlier. It was the only way out, "Oh dear." With burning calves, we eventually reached the top and made the short walk back to our digs. It was at this point that the 'two old farts' in their wisdom decided that they needed an afternoon kip!

A small pit stop of an hour or so, shower and change and then we made our way downstairs to the bar. A rather surreal sight greeted us in the form of a large funeral party, maybe news of our demise had got out! Several 'rattlers' and gin and tonics were consumed and then we finished off the evening with a really tasty meal, a perfect evening.

The following day was less eventful but no less enjoyable. Situated just three miles from our hotel is the beautiful bay of Boscastle. This was the place that suffered massive floods back in 2004. Time really does fly by as I didn't realise that it had been that long ago, not that you could tell now because the local people have done a fantastic job of putting the place back together again. I remember very well the TV news reports at the time, the pictures were truly horrendous and must have been terrifying for all the people that were caught up in the horror of it all. Sian and I found ourselves taking in the whole scene but we struggled to imagine what it must have been really like; it was unimaginable. We carried on doing the tourist bit. We next visited the Witchcraft Museum which had some very interesting artefacts, to say the least! We finished off our visit with the customary cream tea, bloody delicious!

The next destination that was part of our four-day mini-break in Cornwall was the world-famous Jamaica Inn. The main reason we'd booked the inn was because of my long-held interest in the supernatural. The pub has a very long history of haunted poltergeist activity and was a place I'd longed to visit for many years. The inside of the inn has all the features you'd expect to find in a historic old building. Wooden beams, a low ceiling with cosy-logged fireplaces all adding to a really warm welcoming atmosphere. The day we arrived, the weather was blistering hot, so we took advantage of the outside beer garden. A pint of 'rattlers' obviously and a lager shandy for Sian was consumed under the very hot sun.

Now it has to be said that Sian, although she shares some interest in the paranormal, doesn't quite have such a compulsive interest in the subject as me. I think she was feeling slightly nervous at the prospect of staying a night at this haunted location. Adding to her anxiety was the fact that some work colleagues had previously stayed at this location and one person, in particular, had had her foot touched in the middle of the night. When she looked across to her husband, he was fast asleep and was nowhere near her at the time!

After a couple of hours drinking/sunbathing, the 'two old farts' (and there is a common thread here) retired for an afternoon nap. Refreshed and showered we headed to the bar (no, we are not alchies!) Sian was going for it big time; a double gin and tonic was ordered. I got the feeling that she really didn't want to wake up during the night! I had added to Sian's worries somewhat because I'd mentioned that I was planning a small walk-round, an investigation of my own if you like during the night. I really felt that I had to do this whilst we were staying there but Sian was expressing reservations at being left alone at the mercy of the ghosts, so I was experiencing conflicting thoughts. Again we had a nice meal followed by a 'nightcap' Our plan was to take our drinks upstairs and sit on the old bench that was located outside rooms 3 and 4. I knew from watching paranormal programs on TV over the years that these two rooms were the most active for haunted activity.

I personally wasn't worried if I saw a ghost. I was more concerned about how dodgy it may have looked, i.e. myself and Sian sitting outside other people's rooms with drinks in hand looking like a pair of swingers waiting for an invite in! We sat on the bench for a small period of time but it wasn't long before Sian's bravery checked out and we returned to the 'safety' of our room. Whilst lying on the bed, I kept thinking as much as I wanted to go and do my own little ghost hunt bit. I couldn't leave Sian alone in the room, I really couldn't. As a slight alternative, I decided to try and stay awake for the whole night, this was not going to be easy after several drinks and a large meal but I did give it my best shot! I think I lasted to approximately 2 am whereupon my eyes gave up on me. My mind must have still been very active because I kept waking up. This in a strange way was not pissing me off as it usually would. I wanted to be awake so I could make the most of our visit.

However, it wasn't long before something paranormal happened. There was a massive rap on the outside of our window. Thankfully, I was awake at that point but Sian had been woken up by the very loud noise. She asked me what it was. I replied that I wasn't sure but told her not to worry herself about it and to go back to sleep. I had a pretty good idea about what had happened, but I didn't want her to worry. After the knock, I opened up the curtains and looked outside. There was nothing there and it was impossible for anybody to have reached the window without a ladder. I'd forgotten to mention and I'm not making this up. During the evening, a thick veil of fog had descended around the pub from the surrounding moors. This all added to the whole experience as far as I was concerned. It was almost as if it had been deliberately arranged, it looked like a scene from a horror film. I continued to hear some smaller knocks and some creaking floorboards that sounded as if somebody was walking about our room. I couldn't account for this but I was loving it. This was why I was there, to experience paranormal activity first-hand. I made Sian aware about the other noises I'd heard the following morning, I thought it best!

After breakfast, we returned to our room to pack. Now because it was morning, you'd be well within your rights to believe that nothing unusual would happen, well you'd be very wrong! The strangest thing happened as Sian attempted to put her charm bracelet on. She was standing by the side of the bed with her arm outstretched and unfortunately one of the charms fell to the floor. That was the only scientific place it could have fallen but an initial sweep of the area came up with nothing. We both thought that perhaps it had rolled under the bed, a perfectly feasible possibility, but hell no! We still couldn't locate the missing charm. The whole room was turned upside down, both of us were at a total loss, where the fuck could it have gone. Poor Sian had resigned herself to not finding it and suggested that we should mention it at reception as we were checking out. We put the room back to its original state and finished off packing.

At the point of us departing the room, Sian picked up a rucksack that we'd bought especially for our trip. She needed something from it I believe. I need at this point of the account to explain that the said rucksack was on the other side of the room, approximately ten feet away from Sian when she'd attempted to put her bracelet on. At that critical moment in time, the bag was zipped up completely! When Sian opened up that rucksack, guess what she discovered? Yep, you've guessed it. There lying on top of all the other items that were in that bag was the missing charm! Sian shouted out, "How the fuck did that end up in there?" I was lost for words, I really was. It was impossible, there was no way on earth that the charm could have got in that sealed up bag. Sian was obviously very pleased to have found the charm but we both couldn't explain it. It seemed one of the hotels ghostly residents was having a bit of fun at our expense! Bizarre!

In a strange way looking back, it was a perfect going away present from the Jamaica Inn. Were we being thanked for our visit? Perhaps, but I left that old inn feeling very content. It hadn't disappointed, in fact, it had more than lived up to my expectations and I for one can't wait to pay the ghostly hostelry another spooky visit.

On our last day in Cornwall, we planned to visit Bodmin Jail, which was only a fifteen-minute drive from the Jamaica Inn. To say that the jail was a real eye-opener would be an understatement, to say the least. The conditions the prisoners endured were horrific and simply beyond belief, bloody barbaric at best, inhumane at worst. To think it was less than 150 years ago that we treated people like this is quite astonishing. Kids as young as four/five years of age were placed here for what would be considered minor misdemeanours today. Such crimes as petty theft and more often than not, the stealing of food, the poor souls were starving! At the moment there is a huge restoration project happening at the jail. As with some other former jails across the country, it's being turned into a hotel, quite ironic when you think that at one time this would have been the last place you'd have wanted to stay.

Our mini break was now at an end, it had been brilliant and very interesting indeed and I have a feeling that this won't be our last visit to Cornwall. Sian very kindly undertook the task of driving home, but little did I know that my faithful black dog wanted a small walk when I arrived back home.

Oh, fuck!

We arrived home on Friday night and I generally felt Okay, but I started to feel a bit subdued. I put it down to the feeling everyone probably experiences after a break, you know, back to reality and all that. I slept very well that night. I was tired after a very busy four days and I woke up feeling I'd had a good kip. Saturday is my favourite day of the week especially if there is football on, but I was still feeling a bit off colour and I couldn't understand why. This was to carry on during the evening with no improvement in the state of my mood, I was becoming somewhat concerned. I awoke on Sunday morning feeling that my symptoms had got worse overnight.

What the hell is going on?

In my mind, I really didn't want to the think of the worst-case scenario. Was I on my way to another black episode? I reassured myself that it still didn't feel anything like as bad as previous occasions. As I explained in chapter 15, *'The Dog Takes a Nip'*, I was feeling stronger and felt I was able to deal with whatever was going on in a much more controlled manner. No negative thoughts were being allowed to enter my head, which felt quite strange and stranger still was the fact that my 'little demon friend' was not making himself known to me either! This really was all new to me.

Starting to win the war?
Has my demon finally fucked off?
Could I dare to dream of a pain-free life?

But Phil, wait a minute there, mate. My logical side of my brain was telling me that yes, I was making progress, but I still had some way to go. Perhaps for the first time though, I could allow myself to feel confident that I was finally beginning to see the light at the end of a very long tunnel. By Sunday evening I was feeling quite confident that I wasn't going to suffer another episode of 'the black fog'. As I've previously explained, the black clouds normally descend very quickly but this hadn't happened and it didn't feel to me that they were going to. I was slightly confused, but I was very happy, nonetheless. I had a reasonable night sleep and woke up on Monday feeling a lot better, so much, so I managed a workout.

My mind was still trying to make sense of all that had happened over the previous two days. I hadn't suffered

127

another episode nor had I ended up in bed for days on end, which had always happened previously.

I'd won this small battle, now for the war!

I told myself that this could become a common occurrence, that it may take several 'battles' before I eventually win the war against this horrible illness, but I was starting to win and it felt bloody great!

I texted Sian at work later that morning and explained to her that I thought I'd had a small bump in the road, but I was feeling a lot better. She texted back with the words I could tell. Unfortunately, this small episode had left its mark on Sian and she feels rather down. This illness really is a fucking cruel son of a bitch. It takes its toll on not just the sufferer but also your nearest and dearest, it doesn't discriminate. I'm trying to support her the best way I can. Sian for her part is hitting the gym in a bid to get herself out of the black hole. That is all we can both do when negotiating these very tough periods. Although thankfully, there is evidence that there is finally an end in sight.

Now, where is that bloody dog?
It's time he went outside!

Chapter Eighteen
The Demon Drink

It would be a perfectly fair assumption for people reading this book who don't know me to think that maybe I've got a drinking problem. When reading about our 'social adventures' in other chapters of this publication, alcohol is always heavily involved. I would like to take this opportunity to balance out the facts concerning my alcohol consumption. Yes, I and Sian do enjoy a drink at social events but neither of us has a problem with the demon drink. I have never been or even now someone who has felt the need for a pint after work for instance. I could probably count on one hand the amount of times that I've had a drink after work in all of my thirty-seven-year working life. It has never really appealed to me and I use this as my own personal yardstick as to my relationship with alcohol. I'm also not in the habit of drinking in the evenings during the working week either. Since moving to Swindon seventeen years ago, I've driven for a living and so consequently, I would never drink the night before working the following morning. I feel very strongly on the subject of drink-driving and find it wrong on every level. Up to about two years ago (when Sian wasn't working shifts at the hospital) we would go out most Saturday nights. This would be our one night out to let off some steam. Sian works in the nursing profession, so it goes without saying that she invariably needed a drink after enduring all the stress that goes with that job. The stress of the job had, in fact, got so bad that she needed to change jobs. After working at the Great Western Hospital, Swindon for almost ten years, she decided that for the sake of her health and sanity, she needed to look for a new position.

A job at Cirencester Hospital became available and she immediately accepted the job. Her working life is now much more relaxed. The unit she works in only deals in elective day surgery, hence no more shifts or weekend work. Quite horrifying for me personally was the fact that Sian never mentioned to me that on many occasions on her drive to work at the Great Western Hospital, she would be in floods of tears! I only learned of this fact after she had changed jobs and it upset me badly afterwards. The job was literally killing her and I'd said to her on numerous occasions that she needed to leave the hellhole that was the Great Western Hospital.

At that time, I was working as a self-employed courier. Not a job that was as stressful as Sian's by any means, but on a daily basis, I would have to put up with the actions of some crazy muppets, who'd somehow managed to obtain a driving license from somewhere. I was driving crazy distances, 1500-2000+ miles on average every week. And of course, then there was 'London!' I know the city pretty well having grown up on the outskirts of West London but this didn't stop me suffering huge stress when trying to make a delivery in our beloved capital city. With heavy traffic to contend with, high rise office blocks with no 'goods lifts', traffic wardens, the fucking congestion charge and trying to find somewhere to park and deliver. And to finally cap all of this off, you'd be thinking you were parked legally and going about your rightful business only to discover later to your absolute horror that a parking fine had been issued to you by way of a letter that had dropped through your letterbox. All of this would occur because some Gestapo run borough council had decided to install some hidden parking cameras (fucking bastards). Well, you can imagine, in the end, I told the firms I was sub-contracting from that I wasn't prepared any longer to put up with all that crap, so my working trips to London ceased (thank fuck!)

The above circumstances I've just highlighted are the reason why we'd go out every Saturday night. We had to release the pressure valve of life. It kept us both going but little did I know how much it was affecting my underlying health and depression overall. The constant years of heavily working, swimming against the tide more often than not, exercising to stay fit in body and more importantly my mind was taking its toll on me. It went unnoticed for most of the time until I finally would surrender to my illness and would then suffer an episode of the 'black dog'. This situation carried on for many years, vainly thinking that I would eventually drum out my demon, that he'd give up the fight and fuck off but he never did. I sought out professional help many times but nothing ever worked. I thought I was the doing the right thing by soldiering on, trying to be strong for me, for Sian and I used to convince myself that I'd win the war if I just kept going.

It is a well-known fact that alcohol and depression don't mix very well, I've always known this to be true. It's just something I've never paid much attention to over the years.

However, life is short and I don't believe in fully depriving yourself of any vice that you may enjoy. In the last twelve months, I have cut down my alcohol intake considerably, Sian has followed suit. We no longer go out every Saturday night to get smashed, a much more civilised night is now the norm. Quite often we will stay in and have a few beers, maybe a gin and tonic or perhaps the odd glass of red wine now at the weekend (perhaps we are getting old!) But I feel so much better for it.

I'm the last person that can preach to anybody regarding their relationship with alcohol, but I count myself lucky that I'm able to have a drink and then be able to leave it alone for a week or very often longer. When I think back to when my illness began to take a real hold on me some twenty years ago, I could've easily succumbed to the trap of hitting the bottle. It would have been so easy. I'm not a religious person by any means, but I thank whoever it is that is looking over me for guiding me clear of that 'drink self-destruction road'. I perhaps took the road of the two lesser evils, a road that has still been fucking hard. One that has been a constant struggle to stay on at times, but I always believed that the journey I was on was the correct one. This 'road' however, has caused us both to endure so much pain and heartache. We both hoped that eventually, we'd spot the 'white light at the end of the very long tunnel', some hope though! All that regularly used to turn up was that black cloudy fog of depression.

In hindsight though, perhaps I did take the correct road after all. We are both still here fighting, taking on one day at a time and hoping that very soon, I'll get to finally reach the promised land which is located on the other side of that very long dark tunnel of the abyss.

Chapter Nineteen
The 2-Tone Pool Shark!

It was the beginning of August and I had been back home for about a week. Sian and I had already discussed the possibility of a weekend break, so we decided to arrange a visit to Coventry. Coventry! I hear you ask, being 'sent to Coventry' is a well-known expression and you're probably wondering why we'd be so desperate to visit this historical city. To the uninitiated, Coventry is the ancestral home and birthplace of the world-famous 2-tone music. It also happens to be the home city of my all-time favourite group, The Specials, who were, in fact, the early pioneers of the music genre.

In particular, there was one place that I was desperate to visit and the main reason for our trip to the Midlands was The Coventry Music Museum. This place is the mecca, the holy grail of the black and white chequered music phenomenon. It was set up and is, in fact, still run by very enthusiastic volunteers who are welcoming, helpful and above all else, very knowledgeable regarding everything ska/2 tone. There are also two shops selling a vast choice of stock from clothes to all sorts of memorabilia you could possibly wish for. Lastly, I must also mention that on the side is the 2-tone cafe. The grub it sells is exceptional and must be visited. The shops and the cafe operate as fulltime businesses but other than that its volunteer led.

Apart from the very obvious 2-tone memorabilia, the museum also displays artefacts from the late 70s early 80s, These include old TVs, great big video recorders that look absolutely huge now, old furniture, food items and of course all the clothes that were worn at the time. Overall, the museum is a really interesting visit. I was in my element, like a kid in a sweetshop almost. I'd waited a long time to make this visit and I was loving every moment of it. There is a nominal price to pay to gain entry to this wonderful place but it's nowhere near enough I suspect to keep it running as a going concern. I do know that there are regular fundraising events held at the venue, these include live music concerts but they need and deserve much more financial help than they currently receive. I've touched on the above point because, at the time of our visit, we even had trouble finding the museum. Even the local taxi driver was unaware of its location! This I find absolutely disgraceful, to be honest. Now I don't want to appear too disparaging, but when most people think of Coventry, they probably only remember the less glamorous aspects of the city i.e. it was heavily bombed during World War 2 because of its very important and strategic position. Or maybe it's the car industry or perhaps its good old Lady Godiva that comes to mind.

We were to find out after chatting to a member of staff that they receive no help whatsoever from the local authorities, this I find quite scandalous. At the time of our visit, there weren't even any signs to point you in the direction of the museum! The point I'm trying to make is that you would think that the local powers that would embrace and celebrate the very positive image that 2 tone has reflected on the city, but in their case, it seems they're not even acknowledging their previous existence at all!

The positive effect that 2-tone music has had on people like myself stretches from the United Kingdom, Europe, the United States of America and as far away as Asia. It goes without saying that the music genre deserves much more recognition and appreciation in the city of Coventry. Thankfully, the music still lives on, in fact, there has been a massive resurgence of ska bands performing in the last few years and perhaps the best news of all, it's been announced that The Specials are going to tour in 2019 again! Bloody great news! NB. As I go over this final draft of this chapter in March 2019, I'm able to tell you that The Specials are number one in the album charts. Simply incredible. Forty years after they first blasted out their magic sound.

We finished off our visit which involved having our pictures taken holding various instruments. I pretended to play the guitar whilst Sian held a pair of bongo drums in a very suggestive manner (or is that my mucky mind working overtime again!) Next up was a mooch in the two shops, again I was like an over-excited kid. I could have spent an absolute fortune given the chance but instead purchased just a few items. A new trilby hat was bought along with a framed madness, 'The Prince' record and a Neville Staple poster of an upcoming gig at The Assembly Leamington Spa, which I later got framed. Our visit had been bloody brilliant, we both enjoyed the experience very much, but it was now time to head to the pub, which was located very close to our hotel.

The pub in question advertised that they showed sky sports, it was something I'd noticed as we left our hotel on the way to the museum. It was the start of the football season and Jeff and the boys would be bringing us all the news of goals as they went in. I've already mentioned how bad my memory can be these days and the reason for bringing it up again is because sometimes it can be like the blind leading the blind when Sian and I try to remember certain facts. Her memory is no better than mine and as I write this piece, neither of us can remember the name of the pub! When in the process of writing this book, some facts have only come to light when there's been a lot of thought and concerted effort on my part, other facts have literally dropped into my lap as I'm putting pen to paper. All of this I find very frustrating at times. My mind used to be sharp as a tack and remembering dates, facts etc. used to come very easily to me, (oh well, middle age and all that).

Weatherwise the day had started off on a cloudy note and whilst we were at the 2-tone museum, it had literally pissed down, but as we approached the pub, the sun was starting to come out. The pub with no name was huge inside, a big L-shaped bar wrapped itself around the inside of the premises and there were TV screens everywhere you looked. Food was obviously a serious concern for the pub because many people were eating, a sign of the times I suppose. We ordered our drinks and managed to find a suitably placed table that was positioned right in front of the massive main screen (perfect, lovely jubbly). I did treat Sian to a bag of crisps and got a bag of nuts for myself. Well, we both believe eating is cheating, so we wouldn't eat till much later!

The main screen was showing the cricket, which under normal circumstances I'd be happy to watch, but footy comes first in my book and the barman having been asked previously to change the channel to the football had obviously got distracted and forgotten to do this. Finally, he must have heard the mutterings of discontent coming from the locals who had taken their seats around us because the vision is brilliant. Jeff Stelling then appeared on the massive screen. Now the man is certainly no god but to us football fans, he's pretty close, his knowledge of the game is second to none and he hosts the show in a warm and friendly manner. Cracking jokes whenever he can fit them in and only getting slightly flustered when his beloved Hartlepool go a goal down or worse! My team Brentford were away to Sheffield United, who had just been promoted having won League 1, so I felt a draw would be a good result.

The drinks were flowing well, by now the weather was warm, it had turned into a proper summer day and I sat there hopefully waiting for a Brentford goal (some hope!). It wasn't too long before my hopes were dashed though that Sheffield United had scored, we were one down! Half time arrived with no sign of an equalising goal (no change there then!). The second half passes by and no amount of hoping on my part would bring a goal. Oh well, we lost 1-0, but I was having a great time and I wasn't going to let it spoil our day. Sian probably in her wisdom would have said to me "never mind" and I didn't really. We were having a fab day and that day would take another turn when we were approached by one of the local guys who was also watching the scores going in. Problem is, neither Sian nor I can remember his name now either! Bloody annoying.

He was, however, a great chap, very friendly and he went onto say that he was actually a Coventry city fan. He'd stopped attending games along with the many thousands of other disaffected supporters, who were basically protesting at the terrible way the club was being presently run. He commented on my great look. I did look like a throwback to the 1970s, considering everything I had on was ska related. We said that we were visiting his home city for the weekend and had spent the morning at the 2-tone museum. He thought this was brilliant. He'd loved the music back in the day too and said that where we were happened to be very close to the locations was where some of The Specials music videos had been shot. We chatted further on many subjects, but it was to be his agreement with me regarding the perceived lack of appreciation of the music genre by the authorities in Coventry that had struck a chord with me the most.

The drinks kept on flowing and I suspected that Sian was perhaps getting just a little bit bored of the conversation on everything football that my newfound friend and I were having. She was rescued from her ordeal, a friend of the guy we were chatting to came over to our table and asked us if we wanted to play 'killer'. To the uninitiated, this involves a different version of the pool. You all start with three lives and take it in turn to have one shot. If you miss, you lose one life. This process carries on until the last person standing manages to not lose all his or her lives. "Yeah, we're up for that," we said. The organiser of the game took down our names and our entry fee, which I think was £2 each and considering that there were about eighteen to twenty players, the pot was worth winning.

I feel I need to point out that for many years, I'd played pool very seriously. I was captain for a few teams and my greatest achievement was getting my side from league seven to the premier league of our local organisation, the Thames

Valley Pool Association. However, I also need to state that this was quite some time ago and when I could see without the aid of glasses! I don't get much chance to swing my arm these days and although I wasn't by any means the greatest of players, I can more than hold my own when required.

The game started and I recognised a couple of lads straight away that looked like they could play a bit. I had a couple of opening tricky shots, which to my surprise I managed to pot. I say surprise because they were shots that back in the day I'd probably make, but this was now. I was playing with a very rusty arm and wonky eyes! Sian was holding her own too, she was doing ok. A thought did cross my mind at some point that perhaps they'd unwittingly invited a couple of 'bandits' to play and were being 'hustled'. Shots were gradually being missed but I still had all of my lives, I was well in this game, I thought. I was watching my opponents very closely because there's a very common occurrence in 'killer' whereby two players will secretly team up in the hope of sharing the loot. The practice of leaving each other an easy shot is the 'dark art' way of achieving this. It's not hard to spot when this is happening and it fucks me right off, it's not in the spirit of the game I always feel. However, you have to take into account that we were in their pub, their rules, their way of doing things and above all else, we'd been invited to play. I wasn't letting it bother me too much anyway. We were both having a great laugh and we weren't playing for a king's ransom. Sian did very well and was by no means the first player to be knocked out. A few 'bandit' comments were starting to come my way as I kept on potting balls with no loss of lives.

The game had got down to the stage whereby there were two other players and me, pretty soon, one of them got knocked out. The other guy remaining had two lives left and I still had my three. A 50/50 shot was then left for my opponent which he missed, leaving him with just one life. I too was left with a really tough shot next. I hit it well but the ball rattled in the pocket, leaving a really easy shot for my opponent. I knew I was now in a spot of bother. The picture of the game had suddenly changed and not in my favour. He duly potted the easy ball and as expected, left me with a shot to nothing. I was left with what was in my mind, a 30/70% chance of potting the ball. It was a tight cut into the middle pocket, a 'blind cut' they call it. If potting the ball wasn't hard enough, I also had to try and leave the white ball in a safe position so he wouldn't be left with a routine shot. However, my rusty arm happened to be swinging really well that afternoon because I successfully managed to achieve the required end result. He was left with an impossible shot which he missed, meaning the old fart pool shark had mopped up the winnings. We all shook hands and Sian, I and our newfound friend retired to the beer garden to soak up the late afternoon sunshine. Lots more drinks flowed and the conversation got a lot more rowdy as the early evening set in. We were introduced to several more locals by our friend (all of their names escape me now!) but it felt really great to be taken under their wings for the day, they were so warm and welcoming, lovely people! Sian and I both agreed that a return trip to Coventry will be made in the near future.

At some drunken point of the evening, we said our goodbyes and made our way to an Indonesian restaurant that had been recommended to us by the hotel staff. When we arrived, we found the restaurant to be very busy indeed, a good sign that it was as good as what we'd been led to believe.

We were not to be disappointed; the food was the absolute 'dogs' and that view wasn't formed due to the fact we were both wearing 'beer goggles', it really was that excellent. It had proved a brilliant way to finish off our day. It had exceeded all of our expectations, bloody fab.

Thank you, Coventry.

Thank Christ the walk from the restaurant back to our hotel was only very short because this old fart and Sian were two very tired bunnies and we collapsed into our bed with very contented expressions on our 'boats'.

Chapter Twenty

Hanging in There!

Let me be clear from the outset as someone reading this may wonder why I've stuck at my marriage for so long. I love Phil, that's why. Don't get me wrong. I have wanted to leave, no, run in the opposite direction on many, many occasions. I have been asked hundreds of times why I stay. The answer is simple, apart from love, depression is an illness. Would you leave someone who had cancer or any other challenging disease? However, I have learnt to my detriment that this illness is very different, it is unpredictable and has many faces.

In Phil's case, it's selfish, thoughtless, cold and unfeeling. It's painfully difficult to live with someone who appears to despise you, resent you and even hate you whilst carrying the full weight of work, maintaining the house and bringing up a young child. Coping with daily living and being with someone who is severely depressed creates feelings of resentment, guilt, frustration and anger. The hardest part was suppressing all the damaging negative feelings because I didn't want to upset Phil further or hinder any potential recovery. We had no communication, which is damaging to any relationship but in one with the problems we encountered was disastrous.

Somehow, we hurdled from one awful episode to another. Perhaps this made us stronger. I always kept a chink of faith that somewhere in his heart, Phil loved me. That's what kept me going, kept me caring and kept me giving. That was right up until July 2017 when he left. I knew it was coming, I had known for a while. Even during severe bouts of depression where Phil would withdraw, became angry and take to his bed for days at a time, I still believed he cared and I trusted him. Don't misunderstand. I still felt alone, rejected, and somehow it was my fault. Everything changed when I discovered Phil had been deceitful and had messaged other women. That was the beginning of the end. I'm not going to go into depth about the next couple of years because it's too painful and personal, but everything changed for me at the precise moment when I discovered his unfaithfulness. To this day, I don't know if he ever had a physical relationship with anyone but progressively, Phil turned into someone I didn't know anymore.

I watched as he flirted and stared openly at women. We could be anywhere, in the car, shopping, but he was at his worst when out drinking. Alcohol fuels Phil's depression without a doubt. I listened to fountains of abuse about my age, fading looks, my weight and my nagging. I hated going out with him as I knew he would ignore and hurt me. My anxiety levels were through the roof and my thoughts were insane. I contemplated following him, tracking his movements and even looked into hiring a private investigator. I had visions of Phil accepting 'kindness' from his passengers. Phil worked as a cabbie and had once told me in a rage that he was often hit on by younger women. By younger, I presume he meant younger than me!

My 50th birthday came and was almost ignored by Phil. It was then I knew I had lost him. Soon after he announced he wanted to live in Spain, I felt I had been smashed in the face with a sledgehammer. I was angry that I had given and sacrificed so much and it meant nothing. I was also surprisingly relieved because I didn't have to live in constant fear and pain of rejection anymore.

I did everything I could to help Phil with his decision as I only ever wanted him to be happy. Phil didn't move out initially, which was extremely difficult to deal with. He began talking to me as a 'friend', showing me details of villas in Spain, messaging God knows who whilst I carried on cleaning and cooking as if nothing had changed. It was the hardest time of the entire relationship.

Eventually, I asked Phil to leave as it was too painful for me. He didn't seem to care or realise the effect his leaving was having on me. I was dying inside but kept smiling for his sake and that of my daughter, who was obviously worried and also saddened. Phil had been a huge part of her life too. He was after all said and done her stepdad. I helped Phil pack, we sorted out the finances, I saw a solicitor and finally drove him to his brothers where he would stay until he left for Spain. As I dropped him off, Phil thanked me for the lift, turned and walked away. Not a sorry or thank you for the past fifteen years, nothing. I drove home in silence with tears running down my face. I felt I'd failed as a wife, friend and companion.

Phil and I had known each other since school. I always felt that we had something special and were meant to be together. Now that felt like my made-up, stupid romantic notions of fate. Once home, I looked around and saw empty spaces where Phil had been. Our lives in a box somewhere. Stupid memorabilia left behind felt the brunt of my anger and sadness. Fridge magnets bought on the rare holidays we had, china pigs and plants smashed and binned. I drove to Asda and bought new bedding and picture frames for my new start. My scary new life, one without Phil and the pain his illness caused me.

The following couple of weeks helped me to reflect on what had been. I came to the conclusion that it was the depression which made Phil hateful and unfeeling. I determined that he turned his attentions to others because at least he 'felt' something as in his mind, I had become routine and boring. This was not my fault or even Phil's to a degree, it was how the illness had moulded him. Phil's default setting had always been anger. However, I have also realised that having depression is not an excuse to treat others unfairly and I deserve to be happy. My friends were bloody amazing as always. I went to the gym, worked, socialised and was even asked out on a date. Thanks, but no thanks. The next guy I date has to come with a mental health fitness certificate signed by a doctor!

I was just managing to get through each day. I noticed that I wasn't eating an awful lot and gladly dropped a fair few pounds, every cloud! I had asked Phil not to contact me unless he was in dire need of my help. He had attempted suicide on several occasions and I would never turn my back on him. Phil did contact me first asking if I was okay, then to say he was struggling with his decision to leave as it didn't feel right.

I agreed to meet for a chat and decided to let him come home with conditions attached.

There was no way I could allow myself to go back into a destructive relationship that was. If Phil's leaving had taught me anything, it was how wrong our relationship had become and how normal it felt. Well, it wasn't normal, I can see that now. We went on holiday, Phil attempted to work and we tried to repair our destroyed marriage. Before Phil came home, I had to make a promise to myself that I would draw a line under the past and believe in him.

Things were never going to be that simple! After a couple of low periods, Phil agreed to seek help again. He stopped working in October but has been extremely proactive in helping himself. He has been attending counselling sessions and is following a program from a self-help book. We've bought herbal supplements, a lightbox, socialised more and taken long walks together. Since Phil's return, I have had my own very low periods and feelings of depression. I think it's a much-delayed reaction of how bad things were and his leaving. Also, there are still times when Phil's 'old self' returns and I physically feel myself shutdown. I just can't go back there; it was wrong on every level. Marriage should be about love, not hate and resentment.

Depression is not an excuse for a lack of respect, nor should it ever be allowed to inflict constant pain and suffering on the one person who loves you more than anything in the whole wide world. However, I can honestly say that in recent months, I feel very positive about our future. Phil appears to care; we talk and have reconnected. Dare I say, it feels normal, how couples should be.

We have a long way to go, but we are learning to live with this horrible illness. Finally, I still love Phil and that's what matters!

Chapter Twenty-One

Doctor, Beware of the Dog!

While I would never profess to be a real qualified medical professional, my decades of futile struggle allows me to some degree to be ably qualified to pass onto you the reader my very vast knowledge of the horrible illness that is depression. You too may be suffering very badly with this bloody bastard of a monster and you may perhaps recognise similar symptoms as endured by myself in the following pages. I write the following highlighted points in the hope that they may be of some help to you. Depression sometimes allows you to kid yourself that these symptoms are not real even though your brain acknowledges them. Take it from me, they are very real and they need dealing with at the earliest opportunity.

Loss of Interest in Activities You Usually Enjoy

This is a very good flag up, particularly if you find yourself not enjoying things and this happens to turn from perhaps a week, then two/three and then into a month or longer. It was a fact that I eventually noticed in myself. Activities and pastimes that I'd always loved to do, stopped! Not attending football matches was a big yardstick as far as my personal situation was concerned but perhaps a more telling aspect to this point (and the only one that I'd remembered during my recovery) was when I was younger and played football seriously. I'd started to miss matches; I just couldn't be bothered to turn up. The feel-good highs when winning (and this happened a lot as we had a brilliant team) started to diminish and the occasional defeat would leave my mood very deflated and compounded by my early onset of depression.

Other pleasurable experiences also took a hit, sex, (sorry mum) was another thing to hit the deck. My libido nosedived and because I've been on meds for so long, I would go as far to say that my libido has never quite reached the same heights ever since! (Don't worry readers, everything still works very well though!) Other mundane daily activities such as work would suffer too. We all struggle from time to time to lift our head off the pillow in the morning and drag our sorry arses off to work but with depression, this is simply not possible. Again, most people, even if they never like to admit, will take a 'sickie' and the odd day is probably ok. But when one week turns into two and so forth, the alarm bells should be ringing loudly.

Reading, watching TV, everything that most of us do can take a dip or you may lose interest completely in any of the above points. These are all a massive flashing red light and should not be ignored, seek help at once! It goes without saying that the most important factor of all the points I've mentioned so far will and perhaps go unnoticed by yourself but it certainly won't be missed by a partner. This is the very damaging impact that any of the above can have on your relationship. I'm the prime example in all this. I hadn't noticed that the dynamics of my relationship with Sian had changed. My depression hadn't allowed this and I had a very warped view of everything. I would be trundling along thinking we were okay and everything was rosy in our garden but at times I was absolutely wrong to think like that. My fogged-up bonce thought otherwise, however, and all it did was to cause us problems further down the line.

As far as I was concerned, I was putting in all my effort on a daily basis just to function and to do everything what I thought was right. Sian saw things quite differently though. One day, she turned to me and said, "Your depression makes you selfish!" This accusation had never crossed my little mind before and it did knock me back somewhat. I remember getting a horrible sick feeling in my stomach at the time of her revelation. My fucking illness had managed to addle my mind completely.

How the fuck hadn't I know that?

How had I been treating her then?

I was starting to doubt all that I thought I knew about myself!

The point I'm trying to make is that it will almost certainly be your significant other that will notice a change in you, be it your behaviour, your general mood and particularly not wanting to spend time doing things together that had always been enjoyable for you both. It's fair to say that I'm the very last person that is able to preach to anyone regarding my last important point. For so long I just wouldn't open up to Sian. If I had done this earlier, then most probably my depression could have got much needed help a lot sooner, saving both of us much pain and heartbreak. Please, if any of what I've written does resonate with you, you have to try and talk to your other half or perhaps a member of your family. It will be hard but I can assure you of that it won't be anywhere near as hard as it will be if you allow the problem to multiply and fester.

Feeling Down, Sad and Downright Miserable!

The title heading above might seem like a statement of the bleeding obvious when describing how people physically feel when they're in the grips of depression. The words will apply to most people at some point in their lives and quite rightly so. But in most of the cases, the feelings they're experiencing are temporary and will usually dissipate in time. After this has occurred, the person's concerned are able to carry on with their lives as they had been able to do previously. The depressed individual is simply unable to do this. The feelings that they're experiencing can potentially go on for months and even years if the symptoms are not dealt with professionally. These feelings are all tied in with 'enjoyment or lack of' as I explained in my first account and of course it goes hand in hand that if you're feeling bloody miserable, you're not going to want and go out and paint the town red. The problem is though when you're clinically depressed, these symptoms are magnified to a level that is very hard to measure. It will vary from person to person. But let me be clear on this point. It will, however, in most cases totally floor that person. The illness is so debilitating that it shows no mercy to the individual whatsoever. The sheer intensity of the physical symptoms that you have to obligatory endure, I wouldn't wish on my worst enemy. It's indescribable and is a total bitch!

Personally, I always felt like my head was being gripped tightly in a vice during my episodes. It would literally feel as if my head was being crushed. The pressure of the vice, the black fog, it just seemed to go on and on and you never felt like you would get any relief from your ordeal. Of course, eventually, my pain would come to an end and I'd get some blessed mercy thrown my way but it would only be temporary, my black dog always wanted another bite!

So far, I've highlighted what I believe to be two major players that identify whether you may have depression, but there are also other important troubleshooting signs to look out for. These are:

Withdrawal from the People Closest to You

The above-titled heading applied to me personally on every conceivable level. I was the depressed tortoise! It was my default setting. Every time I endured a depressive episode, my head would disappear not inside a shell, but under my duvet cover. This would happen on every single occasion and unbeknown to me at the time it was actually causing irreparable damage to our relationship. Sian was spot on when she'd previously said to me that my depression made me selfish because all I was doing was going into my survival mode each time with little or no thought as to the damaging effect it was having on her. I'm unable to even defend myself on this point because Sian would always say to me once my black dog had eventually fucked off that how she wished that I would talk and share my problems with her. The frustrating aspect for both of us was the fact that 'yes', I did on every single occasion want to talk to her but it was simply impossible on my part. I didn't want to speak to anyone. As

152

crazy as it sounds, my mouth and my conversation with it would totally shut down. It frustrated the life out of me but that is the sheer power of depression.

I could never think rationally when my episodes hit. This was down to the fact that when they did strike, the swiftness and ferocity of my black dog would take me down with little or no warning. I just couldn't stop it once it had decided to hit me on all fronts. This may flick a light on in your own head, perhaps you understand where I'm coming from. Maybe you're stronger than me.

If you find you have the strength to communicate with your nearest and dearest, please try! It will help you so much in the long run. You may also find yourself ignoring phone calls, texts etc., another red light and a sure-fire sign that you're shutting yourself away from the world. I would start taking more and more days off work. I didn't want to face people, which when you consider I was working as a cabbie, did present a slight problem! There were also some occasions when I'd miss an appointment at the doctors, bloody crazy, really! I knew and you know possibly as well that a visit to see a medical specialist was/is a priority. But summoning up the will for these appointments just sometimes seems impossible. And finally, perhaps a very telling sign is the reluctance to want to socialise. I love and still do, enjoy going out but this was the last thing I wanted to do when the black fog descended on me. Some days, I couldn't summon the strength to walk through my front door, never mind surround myself in a pub full of people!

Negative Destructive Thoughts: 'Ruminating'

Let me state for the record right now. I could have been a multiple world champion when it came to the dark art of ruminating. The Usain Bolt of rumination! If there happens to be some poor soul out there that is/was as good as me at overthinking, then you have my total sympathy, my friend. This negative monster possibly contributed more to my depression than anything else put together. The damage that it managed to inflict upon my person cannot be equated, it was a bitch! Over the years I had got to the point of being so good at it that I'd became unaware that I was even doing it! 'Beating myself up' was done on a constant daily basis. Negative and unhelpful thoughts would always enter my mind. I had no weapon to stop them, no constructive way to deal with them. Worst of all, I seemed to thrive and actually enjoy the process of torturing my mind and soul. How fucked up is that?

Very often I'd return from work having had a good day, but you can bet your bottom dollar the only thing my head would concentrate on would be perhaps the one small irritating incident that had occurred during my day. Again, I was just unable to filter out this unimportant issue. It would dominate my thoughts, blocking out all of the good stuff that had happened. It would drive me absolutely mad and I would drive myself insane on occasions. This small 'incident' could have been anything from somebody's inconsiderate driving to some muppet I'd had as a customer. The diagnosis for all of the above is known as 'catastrophising'. Every small negative thought gets blown out of proportion in your head. The worst outcome is considered even when there is no evidence to support what is going on in your depressed addled mind. This form of thinking becomes your default setting and it tends to go totally unnoticed by yourself until it is too late.

This ruminating is a very slow-burn damaging process and it scores very high on the point scoring scale chart that eventually determines the onset of a person developing depression. You may also find yourself blaming everything that bad happens to you on the little voice that you'd often hear in your head that would tell you that your 'worthless, totally useless and a failure at everything you do'. This was something I would hear all the time and eventually you tell yourself that you fully deserve all the crap that happens to you. These thoughts are so self-destructive and serve no positive point whatsoever but a depressed mind can't understand this, it thinks it's normal thinking.

Of course, with a clear mind, it's easy to accept that sometimes 'shit' happens and very often it's not our fault. As I got better, I started to take a reasoned rational approach to problems. I was able to think, *Take it for what it is, Phil*. Give the matter the respect it deserves but don't catastrophise the problem. As you are aware, this was something that previously I was simply unable to do. I've worked very hard in recent months to try and overcome this very hard personal issue. At times, it's been bloody hard but with practice, I'm starting to find it easier to work with. A lot of progress has been made on my part and there is still a long way to go, however, I'm starting to sleigh one of my biggest foes.

I have for the last two months been filling out on a daily basis a 'rumination log'. Everything you do from the point of waking up in the morning until the time you go to bed (not toilet visits, I hasten to add!) is logged. All your activities are written down with a mood score added. Basically, the charts aim to identify your mood and positiveness throughout the day, with any potential dips and low points picked up straight away.

I have found that actively writing everything down has had such a positive impact on my recovery. I'm able to identify right away if there's going to be a mood dip and it's resulted in me being able to deal with it before it can gain any legs and thus cause me any potential damage. It's fair to say that beforehand I was slightly sceptical as regards these rumination logs but for me, they have worked way beyond my expectations. I really believe that they've helped me so much. I ruminate far less than before and I would go as far to say that my war against the bastard demon is coming to an end. I'm quite staggered, to be honest. I was expecting it to take a lot longer to conquer this enemy, but as I've previously stated, the work I've been putting in is nothing like anything else I've ever undertaken before.

Physical Symptoms

One of the main physical symptoms I suffered and still do to a lesser degree is extreme tiredness. Even now as I write this piece some eight months after my very bad breakdown, I still find that I get very easily tired. I'm having more and more early nights, however, on the plus side. I'm feeling better about it. Previously, when going through a depression episode, I would literally spend most of the day and night sleeping and I would still find myself bloody knackered afterwards! This is a major red-light warning and it should definitely not be ignored. Although tiredness is still an issue for me personally, my energy levels are increasing slowly. My gym sessions are starting to become more beneficial as the days pass by but more importantly, they are greatly aiding my recovery.

Other worrying signs to look out for are loss of appetite, weight loss and generally feeling completely run down all the time. It should also be mentioned that the sufferer may have difficulty in sleeping at all. This is in total contrast to my own sleep patterns but nonetheless, it is a very common symptom of depression. A very good way of tracking your sleep pattern is to complete a daily rumination log, as I highlighted earlier. You will find that any changes to your normal sleep cycles will be picked up by you very quickly indeed. My own appetite would always take a nosedive whenever my illness struck. During the first few days of an attack, I would eat or drink absolutely nothing. Even if I'd felt like I needed a drink (which was very often), I just didn't have the energy or the physical will to drag my sorry arse out of bed. Trying to negotiate the stairs when you feel as weak as a new-born kitten would always prove impossible for me. I usually suffered some form of weight loss during these periods but more often than not this would only prove to be temporary.

Everybody, it's fair to say sometimes feels a bit run down. But if you happen to find yourself on the 'purgatory road to despair', these physical symptoms will be of a far more intense nature. For me, personally, apart from the extreme tiredness that I always felt, my body would ache. Ache in a fashion I can only presume that it feels like if you're suffering from flu. Having not (thank God) ever suffered from that particular illness, I can only attest to what other people have told me.

This will cause you to function at levels way below your best. You will find it hard to concentrate on even the most simple tasks. You may think that lack of concentration and loss of functioning doesn't qualify as a 'physical symptom' but I think it does, the brain, after all, is a physical part of your anatomy. One of my biggest enemies, as you are aware, is 'my guilt towards Sian'. I can hear you saying but guilt is an emotion. Yes, you're right, but I do experience physical pain when the guilt monster hits. My stomach will feel like it's tied up in knots, it will feel like a washing machine on fast spin, leaving me wanting to throw up. The sheer intense vice-like feelings that I endure whenever this demon strikes are without a doubt, in my mind, absolutely real and tangible.

Sian will always tell me that I'm far too hard on myself concerning the above. She's right, of course, but my head still doesn't seem able to comprehend that fact, not yet anyway! At the end of the day, no two people's depression symptoms will be exactly the same. However, I need to reiterate that I am by no means medically qualified. But I've given you all of the information regarding my personal experience with this horrible debilitating illness in the hope that you may perhaps identify yourself somewhere. At the very least, my ultimate goal is that it proves to be of some help to you in your own battle with the dark side.

Chapter Twenty-Two
The Good, Crazy Badass Times!

There are, scattered amongst the very dark and debilitating periods that I and Sian have had to overcome, stories that are often downright funny and crazy in the extreme. New Year's Eve 2006 is very fondly remembered. It was to be the very first occasion that we'd meet our long-time good friends Lee and Lisa. Back then they happened to be our new next-door neighbours (well, next door but one if you want to be technical). Sian and I had moved to 'The Ridge' only six months prior and we hadn't been formally introduced to each other. I had noticed them from time to time (no! I wasn't stalking them), but we'd never bumped into each other in the street so consequently, not a spoken word had passed between us.

That situation would change, however, on that fateful New Year's Eve. Sian and I had decided to spend the evening at our new 'local' and so we made the very long walk that was approximately fifty yards to what was to become for many years our second home! The evening started slowly as so often is the case. There also the small matter that I was a stranger in this boozer, not a regular on account on me being new to the area. This wasn't the case for Sian, however, because she had previously drank in the pub when it had first opened, having lived on 'The Ridge' with her first husband (but that's another story).

We hadn't sat down long when I noticed Lee and Lisa walking towards the bar (no change there then!). I remember remarking to Sian that they were neighbours of ours but because she had never set eyes on them, she took me at my word. They sat down on a table next to us, but me being the shy retiring type, hesitated to say hello to them. A few drinks were consumed and maybe an hour or so had passed and we still hadn't made ourselves known to them (we're not normally backward in coming forward). At some point. however, I did notice Lisa looking over in our direction and saying something to Lee. My ears must have been burning because I had this feeling you get when you think someone's talking about you. My physic feelings were proved to be correct on this matter and I've since learnt from Lisa that she'd mentioned to Lee (in her own words), "There's a strange man over there who keeps looking over at us!" (No, I still wasn't stalking them, honestly!) With more alcohol consumed, I finally summoned up the Dutch courage and went over and made our introductions.

The ice was immediately broken, we all joined together and sat on one table. It's very thirsty work when you meet new people in a pub, I mean there is just so much to talk about. Where do you come from? What's your job, interests etc. and most important of all, what football team do you follow! Lee follows Southampton, so he suffers slightly less pain than I do! Although that's debatable! Perhaps you ask about their sexual orientation? Oops! That's a question and piece of conversation for another time! Plenty more drinks and chat were had and the evening played out brilliantly except when it was rudely interrupted at twelve o'clock by 'auld lang syne'. God, I hate that bloody tune, what a load of bollocks!

We were finding our newfound friendship so good that it was decided to carry on our little party back at our gaff. Music was turned on, more drinks poured and a raid into the fridge was made to seek out any much-needed nibbles. Now, there are some defining moments in one's life, be it sober or drunk, that you're able to remember exactly where you were, who you were with and the date of such occasion. 1 January 2007, Lee Kendall, Lisa Bunce (they weren't married then) Sian Gee (we weren't married then either) and obviously my good self-made the rather dubious decision to hit 'the shots'. A strange but true unrelated fact for you: When I and Sian married the following year in 2008, her surname changed from Gee to Green. Nothing unusual about that I hear you say. But in 2007, she qualified as a registered nurse, put the initials R and N into the name Gee and you get Green! Spooky, but true all the same!

Anyway, I digress. Lee in his wisdom had decided to bring along some 'good shit!' Oh dear, I thought, this is going to get very messy indeed! Back then and I still do now for the most part drink mostly beer. Red wine would be next on my consumption list but it usually gives me the hangover from hell if I drink too much of it. I seem to remember Lisa warning us that Lee was always buying this crazy shit, perhaps it stemmed back to his wild days spent in the RAF? I don't know for sure but all I do know is that he still buys various bottles of mental juice to this very day! On this occasion, he'd brought with him two very toxic looking receptacles, one contained a super export-strength port (a drink I absolutely hate) and the other bottle had a label displaying the drink Jägermeister. You have to remember that I grew up in pubs at a time when the only real crazy drink you could order was a snakebite, so the advent of all these super-strength 'shots' you were able to buy were all new to me. I can't honestly remember if Sian had previously partaken in these drinks before or not but I was definitely a 'shots virgin' at that point.

I had witnessed other people when we were out in pubs drinking these 'bombs' and had seen with my own eyes the process of reasonably tipsy happy people then turn into dribbling drunken wrecks. They would stagger all over the place as if they had been hit around the head with a sledgehammer. Unable to put more than two words together, they would be slurring and would then miss their mouth completely when trying to take a further drink from their glass. I even had the odd individual approach me and say, "Hello, mate", them thinking that they must know me from somewhere and I would be thinking to myself, *Who the fuck are you? Piss off, will you?* All of the above had previously resolved my will to avoid these devil's drinks at all cost, that was until Mr Kendall darkened my front door!

Because of the happy occasion and most definitely against my better judgement, I along with Sian decided that we'd have a go at the Jägermeister. Lee poured into the shot glasses what I can only describe as a vile looking green liquid, it looked bloody horrible. It looked like something a military weapons scientist would pour from a test tube and it would likely burn holes in your clothes if you were unlucky enough to spill it on yourself. "You have to down it in one," our newfound friend advised us.

Oh well, nothing ventured, nothing gained, I thought. We all slammed our 'bombs' down. It was fucking disgusting, unlike anything I'd ever tasted before.

"That will give you a good buzz," Lee stated.

What's wrong with that man? I thought. Not only did it taste absolutely foul but it also managed to take off the inside lining of your throat at the same time!

I think Lee was trying to 'sex up' this horrible alcoholic mouthwash. "They're all drinking this at the ski resorts," he exclaimed. I thought to myself that that was the best place for it and preferably thrown over the side of the mountain! The thing was though, Lee had been right. Before very long I was starting to experience 'the good buzz' and perhaps what was more perversely considered by myself and Sian at the time was the stupid fact that we wanted more of this horrid green drink! More 'shots' were had and I for one totally forgot the next hour or so, I was legless! I don't even remember Lee and Lisa leaving to go home.

The next memory that I managed to have was trying to negotiate the stairs. I remember stumbling over at some point, but I eventually got to the top and staggered into the bathroom as I needed a leak before hitting the sack. Anyhow, I found myself standing over the bog trying to point Percy at the porcelain, which was proving very difficult. I was swaying from side to side, backwards and forwards, my head at that point was shot to bits. I was fighting for all my worth just to stay upright. "Fuck! What was in that drink? It's evil, it must be drunk by the devil himself!"

Then it happened! I lost my fight to stay upright and I fell forward face-first onto the tiled shelf that stands behind the toilet. But worst of all I'd managed to face plant the actual sharp edge of this particular shelf with the bridge of my massive conk! I had a deep gash that was over an inch long and there was claret everywhere, what a bloody mess and state to find myself in! Sian called out to see if I was okay but obviously, she didn't receive a coherent reply from me and the next thing I knew was that she was standing in front of me asking me what the hell had I done? To be fair to Sian, I don't think I was making much sense and so she grabbed a towel and tried to stem the heavy flow of blood that was pouring from my nose.

After a while, the bleeding had slowed up enough for Nurse Sian to take a look at my bloodied hooter. "Fucking hell," she cried out, "You're gonna need two or three stitches in that!" I had a large flap of skin hanging over my gash like a loft trap door. Sian moved it back into place to cover the wound and to try and put a stop to the bleeding. Eventually, with lots of pressure applied, the bleeding more or less came to a halt and Sian dressed it as best as she could. This we hoped would hold in case a trip to A&E was needed in the morning. I state the morning because there was no way I was going to the hospital that night. All I wanted to do was collapse on my bed.

Unfortunately for me, the fun and games hadn't quite finished. In hindsight, it probably wasn't the most sensible thing to do, but I attempted to undress myself. At that stage in the proceedings, the safest option for me would have been to just collapse on top of the bed and worry about my clothes in the morning. But as we all know, drink and sensibility don't normally go together in the same sentence. In my drunken state, I hadn't noticed that the wardrobe door was open and when attempting to pull my jeans off, I got one of the legs caught around my foot and so consequently, I fell backwards into where all of my clobbers was hanging up. The end result being me sitting on my arse with all my clothes scattered about my head and on the floor around me. Sian was effing and blinding at me because I'd woken her up, but at the same time, she was absolutely pissing herself at the sight of me blood-soaked, covered in clothes and doing a Trinny and Suzanna in my wardrobe in the middle of the night!

Welcome to 2007, What a Two and Eight!

The next morning, as you can well imagine, we were both seriously hungover. Sian checked my wound, "I think you should go to A&E."

"Naaah! I can't be arsed to go up there at the moment," I remember saying. Even if we'd wanted to go, we couldn't. We were more than likely still over the drink/drive limit. We both agreed that we'd leave it until the following morning and go to the hospital then if it was required. That hospital trip never happened. I came to the conclusion that it would probably heal by itself and if truth be told, I still didn't fancy the potentially long wait at A&E when we got there. The wound did heal eventually, although it probably did need a stitch or two, but contrary to popular belief, us southerners are made of sterner stuff. The scar on my nose has faded with time but that great nightstick in the mind for all sorts of different reasons. Our great friendship with Lee and Lisa began on that eventful evening and is still going strong to this very day.

Thank you, Lee and Lisa, we both love you.

But leaky, you can stick that Jägermeister where the sun doesn't shine, my good friend!

The great city of Cardiff has featured very heavily in our lives ever since we hooked up with 'the good doctor, Andy Davies'. This has caused us to make many trips along with the M4 into Wales and so consequently, we've had to endure many hungover trips back home into England afterwards. Sporting wise, Cardiff hasn't been very kind to me. On the two occasions, I'd been to what was called the Millennium Stadium. I'd witnessed my football team Brentford lose both games. On our numerous trips to the capital city, we've never actually physically attended a Rugby International, preferring to watch the game in one of the many city-centre pubs has always been the outcome. Our plan is to make sure Wales are always playing at home and preferably against England. On these home occasions, the city of Cardiff is literally besieged by what seems half the population of Wales. The place is absolutely jammed and a sea of red Welsh replica shirts is all that you can see before you, it's a pretty amazing sight! A few token white England shirts can be spotted from time to time but they're definitely in the minority.

You may come to the conclusion that these few crazy souls bravely wearing the red rose must be complete bonkers. But that is the brilliant difference between football and rugby. The atmosphere is always highly charged, everyone is up for the match but I've never witnessed a hint of trouble ever. Unfortunately, I'm unable to say the same thing regarding football. I had the misfortune to witness many times in the late '70s and early '80s the scourge that is football hooliganism. Thankfully as we all know, this problem doesn't exist in this country on that scale any longer. But even today when I attend football games, I sometimes find the atmosphere to be somewhat hostile between opposition supporters. This is something that doesn't seem to happen at rugby matches. Lots of good-natured banter will be exchanged between the two sets of fans but it's never malicious, it's always done in a friendly fashion. For reasons, I will go more into detail later, we now stay away from the city centre.

A favourite local hostelry of Andy's is called 'The Claude'. It's a great pub, very large with plenty of TVs and a large screen to boot! Because of all this, it's a great venue to enjoy a beer or two whilst watching the big game. The locals are also very friendly, which for reasons I'll explain is a good thing. On one of our more recent visits to Cardiff, Wales were actually playing 'away' against England at Twickenham. But this didn't stop us wanting to pay 'the good doctor' a visit anyhow. We knew the crack would be good and the atmosphere and copious amounts of drink would result in much frivolity.

On this particular excursion to Wales in March 2016, we found ourselves in The Claude. The pub was rammed, again a wall of red shirts enveloped the surroundings and amongst all of this backdrop sat one very lonely looking Englishman, proudly wearing his white shirt. As far as I could tell, apart from my good self (who wasn't wearing any colours), we were the only two English people in the whole pub. However, I was to be proved wrong on this point. At some point before the game got underway and whilst taking a large glug of my beer, a rather strange sight came into my view. What I saw made me nearly cough up my beer. Walking past me was a chap wearing a full set of armour dressed as though he was St. George himself! It was a surreal sight and one of those occasions when you think your eyes are betraying you. Once you realised that the sight before you was real, the whole scenario became absolutely hilarious. Talk about walking into your enemy's back yard with no weapons to aid you!

The thing was that he didn't need to defend himself. In fact, his only problem was trying to fend people off so he could reach the bar and buy himself a drink. Everybody wanted to stop and chat with him, to have a laugh and he even found himself in numerous photographs with Welsh supporters, it was brilliant! A small miracle even happened on that day; England managed to win the game. This didn't change the atmosphere in the pub one little bit though. People sitting near our table had deduced the fact that I too was English (maybe it was the cheering that gave me away!). But they came over and we shook hands, we talked and joked and had plenty of banter. I was even offered a drink on countless occasions. God, I love the Welsh folk!

The reasons for our not venturing into the city of Cardiff on international match days will become very apparent to you as you read the following pages. There are two very notable occasions that occurred in Cardiff that'd helped us come to our final decision. The first account goes all the way back to February 2009. The purpose of our visit was to have a catch up with Andy but we were also going to be watching a game that involved an odd-shaped ball. At that time, we always made our way into the city centre. We would go in mainly because the atmosphere in the city on matchdays is positively electric, it causes your hairs on the back of your neck stand up, it really is brilliant! The city was full of rugby fans that had come from all over Wales (and a few brave souls from England!) Andy informed us that the valley is empty out on these occasions and you do get the impression that the half the population of Wales is in attendance. Many of these revellers will spend the whole weekend absolutely determined to have a great time. This will normally involve drinking, singing, chips and kebabs, although not necessarily in that particular order!

We frequented several pubs in our search for a suitable venue that housed a big screen and eventually our efforts were to be rewarded. Upon us walking into this boozer, we were met with the sight with what I can only describe as an 'absolute wall of red'. Just about everyone was wearing the red shirt of Wales and that included the bar staff. Flags with the Welsh dragon on were draped from every vantage point and all sorts of Welsh paraphernalia was on display. This included blow up leeks and most funny of all, blow up sheep! (You've got to admire their sense of humour!) There was no sign of an Englishman anywhere (except for one very stupid sod!). The beers flowed as quickly as the game seemed to pass by and Wales won again! There was to be no cheering from this very quiet Englishman, just lots of polite clapping and besides I'd got very used to being on the losing side in Cardiff, be it football or rugby at that particular point in history.

Towards the end of a long day and evening of drinking copious amounts of alcohol, I think one of us decided that we needed something to eat. We found ourselves walking down Cardiff's famous 'chip alley'. To the uninitiated, this street is a junk food addicts idea of heaven. Virtually, every single building is a take-away of some description and the vendors there must make a small fortune at weekends and especially so on international matchdays. You can literally feel your arteries clogging up as you walk past the various shops selling fried chicken, elephant leg kebabs on spits, Indian snacks and of course, mountains of greasy chips.

I seem to remember that we grabbed a portion of these greasy chips just to keep us going, but what we really wanted was 'a ruby'. It was getting late but Andy said he knew of one Indian restaurant that always stayed open late than the rest. Sian and I were more than happy that we'd be having a ruby. We're absolute 'curry heads'. We more or less live on the grub, we just can't get enough of 'the burn'. The three of us were walking (no we weren't, we were staggering very badly!) for what in our drunken minds seemed like ages. Eventually, we arrived at the curry house (its name obviously escapes me now). It was very busy still, always a good sign as to how good the establishment is. However, we were in luck; there was a table waiting for us.

Andy is quite an aficionado when it comes to seeking out a good curry. You know you gonna get a good meal when it's a restaurant of his choice. He'd done us proud again. The meal was excellent and even after a day of heavy drinking I could attest to this, years of practice, I suppose! A suggestion was put forward by somebody that we should try and phone a cab. One of the waiters said that they would bell a company they always used. This seemed a good play. However, he informed us that there was a forty-five to sixty-minute wait. Apparently, it was very busy (something to do with an international rugby match being played earlier we were told). *No shit sherlock*, I thought to myself!

The restaurant wasn't due to close until 2:30 am and after checking the time, I discovered it was only 12:45 am. We wondered what we were going to do to fill the time, it was a bitterly cold night and none of us fancied having to stand outside in the freezing conditions for too long. Thankfully, the manager of the curry house said that it was okay for us to stay inside on the condition that we bought another drink. (Hey, I like those conditions!) Even though we were all stuffed with curry and had had more than enough to drink, buying another round of drinks really was a no brainer, it was far more preferable than standing outside in the near arctic conditions. Sian was 'very tired' (pissed as a fart more like) by this point. Andy definitely was, he was fast asleep with his head laying on the table, dreaming of a Welsh try or something similar. I was knackered too and was most definitely the worse for wear, it had been a very long session.

Well over an hour had passed and I got a member of staff to call the cab company again. The waiter was informed that the wait was still at least another forty-five minutes. "Oh shit," I groaned, all I wanted was my bed, not another beer! Andy had woken up from his drunken slumber and was totally confused as to his whereabouts. "Are we home yet?"

"Are we home yet?" I exclaimed as I repeated his question. "We're still in the curry house, you daft plonker!" I think it's fair to say that we'd all reached the point where we were getting a bit agitated, we all just wanted to hit the sack! Another thirty minutes or so passed and still no sign of the bloody cab.

"That's it, I've had enough of this. I'll get us a fucking taxi," Sian said. With that announcement still ringing in our ears, she stood up and marched towards the exit door. She stood by the large window outside and we both wondered what was going to happen next. I wasn't too happy for her to be stood outside alone so after a while, I decided that I'd join her in the cold. I told Andy that I was going outside with Sian as I didn't want her being on her own at that time of night. The problem was that by the time I'd looked away from Sian

171

to tell Andy all of this and me looking back, she'd disappeared! *Fuck, where's she gone*, I thought.

I didn't need to worry though. By the time I got outside the restaurant, Sian was running back towards me and shouting, "Come on, I've got us a cab!"

"What the fuck," I replied, "How did you manage that?" She didn't say and at that moment in time, I didn't really care, to be honest. Andy was called and we all jumped in the cab to head off home. As you can imagine, I and Andy were desperate to find out exactly how she'd managed to commandeer the taxi. "Come on then, tell us how you did it then?" I enquired. It turned out that she'd been flashing her boobs at a few passing empty cabs! Andy and I hadn't been able to see this from inside the curry house so were completely unaware of her antics. She stated that the third or fourth car had made the decision to stop, which was just as well, it was a very cold night after all!

She explained further that our poor driver had nearly written his car off at the sight of Sian's ample charms. "He skidded right across the road, it was lucky there was no car coming in the opposite direction," she pointed out. We were absolutely pissing ourselves laughing during the entire journey back to Andy's house. It was just so funny; my sides were literally aching! I really shouldn't have been too surprised by Sian's tactics; she's always been a very resourceful kind of girl!

Hopefully, by this point, you're starting to draw a picture in your mind regarding the phenomenon that is the elusive and very rare international matchday Cardiff taxicab. We know this fact to be true. We've spent time in Cardiff at other so-called normal times when getting a cab is no problem

172

whatsoever. It's only fair to say that on most occasions the cars have been very punctual with little or no wait at all. At various times, we've attempted to find the answer to this problem by asking cab drivers why so many of them won't work when the rugby is on. The replies we receive are always fairly similar, "There's no point, it's too busy, it's not worth the aggro trying to get around the city." I can hear the cogs in your mind working as you're trying to fathom out those startling statements of fact. Too busy! I hear you ask.

We would counter this by saying that it must be worth working still, surely! "No mate, it takes too long to complete a job." Again we'd point out that there would be possibly hundreds upon hundreds of people such as us that would need a cab at some point during the evening. The reply we got was always the same. "It's still a no my friend, I prefer not to work on matchdays."

Perhaps I need to enlighten you if you've never found yourself in Cardiff during international rugby matchdays. I can empathise with the cab drivers to some degree. As an ex cab driver myself, I know only too well how frustrating it can be to get stuck in heavy traffic going nowhere fast. It's fine for the Hackney cabs because their metres run continually but a private hire driver earns his money on mileage. So, when you're sat in a queue, you're consequently not earning much money. Anyhow, I digress.

Cardiff on these special occasions is just so busy, the place is an absolute madhouse. There are throngs of people everywhere you look and they're coming and going in all directions, mostly moving from one watering hole to another. Outside of these pubs, you will find queues of people trying to gain entry but their way in will be blocked by big burly but nearly always very friendly bouncers. The police and the local authority's actions further compound the problem for the city's cab drivers. However, the closing off of certain major streets within the city centre is a necessary precaution. There are just too many people milling about and the roads are needed and used as pavements. This situation carries on all evening and into the early hours even though the match has finished several hours before.

Friday 6 February 2015, the date of yet another eventful weekend spent in the Welsh capital city. I'm more than happy to be corrected on this point but the above date was to be, I think, the first time that a six nations game was to be played on a Friday night. Sian and I left Swindon around midday on that momentous day. It's a relatively short drive and it normally only takes around one hour and twenty minutes to reach Andy's house. The weather was lovely and the sun was shining as we made our way along the M4 towards Wales with both of us very much looking forward to a great weekend spent with the 'good doctor'.

We'd reached as far as Bristol when all of a sudden, the traffic came to a grinding halt. I didn't worry about it too much as I was more than familiar with Bristol's heavy traffic, especially at the junction of the M5. I just thought it would clear pretty quickly as it usually did. Unfortunately for us, we'd had the CD playing, so we'd missed any traffic reports on the radio and what was more strange was that there hadn't been any warnings on the matrix signs either. The only conclusion we could come to was that the queue had literally only just started! You know you're luck's out when just at the precise moment you switch the radio on, some woman tells you over the airwaves that there's very heavy traffic at the junction of the M4/5 and M32 at Bristol! (We bloody know, we sat in it, you daft mare!)

Worse information was to come from our very helpful traffic reporter. She went onto say that the traffic from our junction was moving very, very slowly all the way along the M4 into Wales until it reached Cardiff! "What the fuck?" I and Sian uttered in unison. We couldn't understand why the traffic was so bad. I mean we'd done that journey on countless occasions previously when the rugby was on and the heavy traffic had never been that bad. It really did turn into a slow, painful and torturous drive. It was simply impossible to build up a head of steam, the motorway was absolutely clogged up. Eventually, we arrived at Andy's house, the journey had taken close to four hours!

We kept in constant contact with Andy and it was decided that he and his then-wife, Gemma, would head off into Cardiff to find somewhere suitable to watch the game and we'd catch up with them as soon as we could. By the time we arrived, we both needed a toilet break and a drink but not necessarily in that particular order! I took the liberty of phoning the cab company in advance and hoping upon hope that we would arrive at Andy's before the cab turned up. Thankfully, this was achieved, although it had been a very close-run thing. The taxi turned up just after we had pulled up at Andy's, phew! Out of one car, we jumped and then jumped into another and off we went, still busting for a piss and desperate for a beer. The cab dropped us off at the closest possible point, the major streets had already been closed off by the police. Cardiff was busier than normal if that was even possible. It was rammed full of people already having a great crack. At this point, it's worth noting that there was still nearly three hours to kick-off and yet the place was already bouncing off the walls, it was simply incredible.

We eventually found the establishment that Andy and Gemma had chosen (déjà vu here, I can't remember the bloody name of the pub again!). We said hello to the already stationed bouncers and made our way inside. Fucking hell! trying to locate our friends was going to be easier said than done. You could hardly move; the place was like a sardine can and I was slightly worried for Sian as she gets a bit uncomfortable in packed enclosed spaces. There wasn't so much as a sea of red in this gaff, it seemed to be more of a neutral venue and as we fought our way through the crowd, you could spot plenty of white England shirts being worn. Some people seemed intent on impeding our way, they just wouldn't move. They received the broadside of my shoulder, not something I'd do normally, but this wasn't a normal situation and besides, by this point, I and Sian were on the verge of wetting ourselves!

Thankfully, Andy and Gemma had spotted us first, maybe they'd heard the commotion going on behind us. I'm not sure now, to be honest, we were just glad to have found them. We said hello as we rush past them. I had located the bogs and we both ran down the stairs like our life depended on it, leaving Andy and Gemma with a rather bemused look on their faces!

With the python siphoned so to speak and with Sian also blissfully relieved, we were then able to say hello properly. Lots of hugs, kisses and so forth followed, then, perhaps best of all, drinks were ordered. Andy explained the reasons as to why Cardiff was even busier than normal. Apparently, extra Welsh supporters had decided to descend on the capital city, as they were expecting to do in what was Andy's own words, "Give the English a damn good thrashing!"

Oh dear, I thought. To be fair, it was a perfectly valid assumption for the home supporters to reach. After all, this had happened two years prior the last time England had visited Cardiff in the six nations. On that occasion, the Welsh had battered us 30-3 and yes, you've guessed it, I was in Cardiff for yet what was another painful losing sporting experience! (Why do I keep visiting this place?) Andy was right though. It did seem as though the Welsh world and his wife had deserted the valleys in anticipation of giving the English a good kick up the arse! I also think that the fact the match was being played on a Friday night had been a factor in swelling the crowd, it was after all an extra night on the lash for the party-loving Welsh fans. Sian made the comment that the extra traffic on the M4 earlier could have been down to the fact that there were definitely more England fans in attendance. I think she was probably right on this occasion. After lots of conversation and drinks, the game finally started.

Within a couple of minutes, Wales scored a try. *Oh no*, I thought, *here we go again!* My heart sunk; I really couldn't stomach another heavy beating. Memories of two years prior flooded my mind and it didn't feel good, in fact, I feared the very worst! I love the city of Cardiff, but at that time, I was beginning to get sick and tired of nearly always coming off second best, I really was! *Oh well, such is life*, I thought. At least I was in good company enjoying a drink, it could've been worse, I suppose. However, to my pleasant surprise, England started to raise their game. The only predictable thing about sport is its unpredictability, that's why I love it so much. The unthinkable had happened and England had managed to take the lead. Fucking hell! I wasn't expecting that at the time, I can tell you. I was even experiencing feelings that were strangely alien to me whilst watching matches in Cardiff. It felt good for a change and it left me with a nice warm feeling inside.

The England fans in the pub were making their voices heard, they were very noisy and lots of good-natured banter was exchanged between the rival supporters. The atmosphere was positively electric! The final whistle was blown by the referee and England had prevailed and won the game 21-16. It was at this point that I knew a good night was about to follow for this one very happy and relieved English fan.

The beers seemed to flow all the more easily during the rest of day/evening and of course, it goes without saying that they also tasted a lot sweeter because of England's win. Although I'm not the biggest of Rugby fans and some of the rules still leave me somewhat baffled to this day, I do enjoy the six nations and of course, the rugby world cup. My interest in the game has definitely grown ever since I hooked up with my 'Welsh wife'. So for anyone reading this who knows me as just a football nut, it's down to her as to why I now take an interest in the odd-shaped ball game! As we crawled from pub to different pub, I felt like the Ready Brek kid. It was freezing, but I had this lovely warm feeling inside of me and perhaps I was glowing orange on the outside too!

We even took the precaution of phoning several taxi companies much earlier than we normally would. We didn't want to get caught out again but the signs looked a bit ominous. Waiting times of between one and a half to two hours were being quoted. (Oh no! Not this situation again was what was going through all of our minds.) What was compounding the issue further was the very cold weather. In fact, I'd go as far as to say that this particular February evening was positively Baltic. The cold wind was literally cutting us in half and there was also the fact that we all had alcohol in our systems, which was making us feel the freezing conditions even more.

Andy suggested that it might be a good idea to wait and queue at one of the many taxi ranks that are dotted about the city. It seemed the most sensible thing to do and even if our fare home was going to be potentially a little bit more expensive. We were certainly not worried about that small matter at the time. We chose to stop and queue at a rank that Andy had successfully used previously and one that he thought was a good option. The rank was situated outside the Hilton Hotel, a fact that didn't seem too important to us at the time. Well, we waited and waited; every now and then, an empty cab would pass us going the other way but absolutely none appeared coming in our direction! (This was bonkers. What the hell was going on?) Andy tried to reassure us that we were going to get a cab soon. Apparently, we were waiting at one of Cardiff's main taxi-ranks, but at the time, I felt there was more chance of spotting a group of god loving nuns out on the lash, then there was us managing to hijack a cab!

I hope by now you're becoming more aware of what is known locally as 'the lesser spotted Cardiff taxicab'. This particular beast is a very rare phenomenon indeed on rugby international dates. There is even a local legend that says many cabs often disappear when they head off into the valleys with their punters and are never to be seen again! (or maybe I just made that story up). But you could well believe that tall tale that evening. There didn't seem to be much hope of us getting home by any means other than walking but this too was out of the question. We'd been queuing for about an hour and we were both frozen to the bone and I wanted to get Sian out of the cold.

I've already mentioned that we had found ourselves standing outside the Hilton Hotel. We'd noticed people going in as we were queuing but hadn't given the matter much thought. We just thought they must have been residents of the hotel. I said to Sian that we might be able to get a drink and hopefully stay there until the crowds die down somewhat. As we made our way inside, we were met with a rather strange sight. There were people everywhere, some were waiting to be served at the bar, others were standing. There were also people sitting on the chairs and floor of the lobby and it looked as though people were using what looked like a conference suite also. Everyone appeared to have a drink and we were told by the bar staff that as long as we used their services, we could stay inside for as long as we wanted. The management in their divine wisdom had made this decision as they'd got wind of the desperate situation that was happening outside and in fact all over the city.

Andy and Gemma made the decision to walk to another but hopefully less busy taxi-rank. They would keep us informed as to the situation and would come back to collect us if successful. It really felt quite strange, perhaps what it feels like when you've been asked to evacuate your home? Some people were literally crashed out, probably as a result of a good time on the lash. Others had formed groups and were laughing and joking at the situation we had all managed to find ourselves in. It was a bizarre situation and one I will never forget. Thankfully, however, we were in the warm at last and were thawing out. The cold really had penetrated our old bones that night! We found a vacant spot on the floor, it wasn't ideal, but at least we had a wall to lean against. Both of us had reached the point where we'd had enough to drink really and the excesses of the day were beginning to take their toll.

In our younger days, we would have carried on with the merriment until the break of dawn but those days are long since gone and both of us were well past our 'best before date'. I started drifting off to sleep but would often wake up with a jolt. My subconscious mind was probably telling me that I shouldn't be kipping in a hotel lobby and that I should really be sleeping soundly in one of the rooms above. After about an hour or so, Andy texted Sian to inform us that they'd given up waiting for a taxi and had started the long very cold walk home (brave souls). At this point, Sian started to phone the various cab companies once more, but the situation hadn't changed whatsoever. There was still on average a two-hour wait and we really did think that the rest of our night was going to be spent on that hotel lobby floor.

More drifting in and out of sleep was to follow until Sian woke me to give me some good news. It seemed salvation was at hand. Andy had messaged Sian once more and apparently, he and Gemma were in a cab and they were on their way back into Cardiff to pick us up. We really didn't expect to hear from Andy again, to be honest. It was quite feasible that they could've been near if not home by the time that he got back to us. However, his messaged words were literally music to our ears, but we did wonder at the time how he'd managed to grab a cab. There was to be no topless drama on this occasion, just good old-fashioned luck. Andy had waved a car down apparently, who just happened to be heading back into the city anyway, so the driver received a Brucie bonus for his troubles. Before very long they'd pulled up outside the Hilton Hotel. We were waiting by the entrance because we could see the street and it meant that we didn't have to stand and wait outside in the cold.

As we made our way towards the taxi the commotion that was starting to manifest in front of us was quite astonishing to say the very least. Andy had got out of the car and was holding a door open. This would hopefully signal to wait and pass people that this cab was very much spoken for. They obviously took no notice of Andy's actions or more to the point, they were probably just so desperate to get a ride home as well. He was literally having to push people away and screaming at them to piss off!

To me it was pretty evident that these poor people were not interested in speaking to the driver, they just wanted to nick our cab! I grabbed hold of Sian's arm and I put my mean face on, there was simply no way we were going to miss out on this much-prized cab. I marched towards the car whilst holding hold of Sian's arm very tightly because this situation had the potential to turn very nasty. I had to body check a few people out of the way and others received a push aside until I finally managed to get Sian in the car. It was pure mayhem. I still had to get inside this bloody cab and more jostling, lots of swearing and the occasional punch on the nose by my good self were to follow until I eventually made it inside the cab. The poor driver, bless him, was shitting himself. He must have wondered what he'd done to deserve all of this trouble. The funny thing was that once we were all inside, we were actually finding the whole situation bizarrely hilarious. I kid you not, there were bodies and limbs draped all over this cab, it could have been a film scene from the *Zombie Apocalypse!* Our driver pulled away from the scene with bodies falling off all over the road, it was fucking insane but very funny to us in our intoxicated state!

We eventually made it back to Andy's at about five in the morning. Looking back at the event now, it was just another one of those crazy nights in Cardiff. Every time we go there, something daft seems to happen and I've only told you a few tales of our exploits in that great Welsh city. You can fully understand the reasons why a ten-minute walk to The Claude pub is now our much-preferred option. We are able to stagger back to Andy's without having to worry about hiring that very rare beast, 'the lesser spotted taxicab'.

Chapter Twenty-Three
The End in Sight!

Sessions 15 and 16

My visit to Bradford House for session 15 in June 2018 was for all intents and purposes the second review of all the previous appointments I'd shared with Isobel. The session was a very much welcomed lighter affair for me. The extreme tiredness had lessened slightly to some degree, but I was still feeling the effects of my recovery and it was still an ongoing daily battle to function at the levels at what I considered to be normal. I clarified to Isobel that I felt happy and very relieved that we'd covered and indeed exhausted all the important relevant issues. The whole process had very been traumatic and without any shadow of a doubt had been the hardest feat that I'd ever accomplished. I was and very much still am very proud of this achievement. I quite often take a step back and wonder just how I'd managed it, to be honest. I mean, at one time I couldn't even muster the strength to lift the duvet cover off the top of my head. Never mind taking on all of my demons in a full-scale war.

A two-week break followed and session 16 on the 4 July found me in a rather philosophical frame of mind. "Hello,

Phil, it's good to see you again," Isobel remarked. She always said this at the beginning of our get-togethers and it always resulted in reassuring me that what was to follow was all going to turn out ok. My state of mind had come about because as I explained to my lovely counsellor my handling of my thoughts, particularly when it came to damaging negative one, it was continuing to be processed and dealt with much more positively by my brain. An example of this is best illustrated by the rather troubling thoughts I was still receiving regarding my seventh and final suicide attempt. As I've previously highlighted, the date of my seventh attempt coincided with our wedding anniversary, not a very good choice of dates to put it mildly! It had and still was giving me cold sweats whenever it crossed my mind, which was way too often for my liking. On a much more positive note though, I explained that these horrible intrusive thoughts were not dragging me down, I just wasn't allowing it to happen.

"There's no doubt, Isobel, these thoughts would've pulled me down into the murky depths of despair before I started my recovery. I have no qualms in stating that fact."

Obviously, I was ecstatic at the progress that was being made, but along with those nagging thoughts, I was still getting and what with my own ingrained slightly pessimistic nature, I had to explain that there were still times that I doubted myself. "But why do think along those lines, Phil?"

"The sheer length of my illness, I suppose, the deep-rooted problems were never going to disappear overnight, far from it!" There was also my well documented medical history that hadn't been available to me until very recently. This was perhaps one of the main reasons why I wasn't 100%

convinced in my mind that I wouldn't fall victim to depression again at some point in the future.

"You have come a very long way, Phil, in a short space of time, cut yourself some slack." Those words coming from Isobel were said in a manner that almost sounded as though she was giving me an order, but she was right and more to the bloody point, I knew that fact already! It's just sometimes my fog-clearing mind forgets this point and needs a kick up the arse periodically to give it a gentle reminder!

The fact that my depressed addled head was now in recovery mode was making me question all of my long-term held beliefs. "I'm having to learn everything again, Isobel."

"What do you mean, Phil?" Isobel had a rather quizzical pained expression on her face and I had to clarify to her exactly what I meant regarding the statement I'd just made.

"I'm having to make sense of everything. I'm questioning all of my belief patterns all of the time." A short pause followed. "For so many years, my depressed head had in its own way made all of my conscious thoughts seem real to me and I didn't know any different."

"Do you find that a bit confusing then, Phil?"

"Yeah, I do. The way I think about certain subjects has changed. I'm not so cynical, but that doesn't mean I've stopped shouting at the TV at times, it's just certain things feel slightly different to me now and it feels very strange." Even before our session, I'd found myself wondering many times if this new way of thinking was new or was it the 'old Phil' re-emerging? I was finding it a bit disconcerting at times because the illness had been a part of me for my whole adult life, so consequently, I wasn't too sure who the normal Phil was!

All of this was affecting me, but not in a damaging way. The uncertainty of my thoughts was actually making me somewhat impatient. That might seem a bit crazy to you, but I just wanted confirmation that what I was beginning to think and believe in my swede was actually a new concept, or dare I say, the 'old Phil' returning. An example of my impatience had surfaced earlier in the week. Sian always receives a daily text at work from me. It's just a quick few lines to ask if she's okay, is her day going well etc. On that particular day, I expressed my frustrations to her in a message that said: "I don't feel like I'm getting anywhere, my recovery has stalled!"

"How bloody stupid is that?" I said to Isobel. "What the hell was I thinking? Was I having an off day? Yes, Phil, that was probably all it was, don't worry yourself too much about it," came my reply. Of course, I knew only too well that my perceived worries in relation to my recovery were simply unfounded, but this was the daily battle I was facing at the time. Sian, brilliant and supportive as always, replied to my text with all the reassuring words that I needed.

"Phil, sometimes you're a right bonehead!"

There was also another small matter I needed to get off my chest. I was slightly concerned that my dialogue with Isobel was going to soon dry up. We had after all covered all of the major issues on a very exhaustive basis and I didn't feel the need to go back and visit those very traumatic circumstances once again. I went further, explaining that I felt that I'd reached the point where I didn't think that weekly counselling sessions were required and perhaps there were by now other people that were in desperate need of their help. I was more than happy to give up my slot. I felt that it was time to stop or at the very least cut right back on my sessions. Isobel would need to check with Barbara (manager) about the situation as it was not clear how we would go forward on this issue. However, I was quick to point out that I was very keen to 'stay in the loop'. I didn't want to cut all ties with this wonderful organisation in case I suffered a wobble in the future.

Isobel then went on to make a very good point. She highlighted the fact that my depressive symptoms were at their worst during the autumn/winter months. This time of year also coincided with many of my suicide attempts, so she really did have a valid point. We both agreed that perhaps I should carry on with the sessions periodically at least, for the time being, just to see how I dealt with the onset of the autumn/winter blues. This situation was going to have to sit on the back burner for three weeks though due to Isobel going away on holiday. However, the positive side to all of this meant that at least I would get a much-needed break and it didn't arrive a minute too soon!

Chapter Twenty-Four

Russian Roulette:
Vodka and Pain – Part 1

I have a confession to make. I really hadn't given any consideration to include in this book the subject of the Russian 2018 World Cup. As you are now well aware, my undying love for the beautiful game simply can't be measured in words. England's recent tournament performances which can only be best described as absolutely woeful were the main reasons that I hadn't given the matter any serious thought whatsoever. A quick glance at the outside of my house at the time would have given you a clear indication as to my own very low expectations of the national side prospects in Russia.

I state the above because normally, my house would be adorned with flags, bunting etc., but this time around, I just hadn't bothered to hang up any of my patriotic colours. I think a large percentage of the English population shared the same damming opinion because I'd never seen such a lack of England paraphernalia, be it hanging from people's properties or cars and vans. You could've been forgiven that England hadn't even qualified for what is arguably alongside the Olympic Games, the biggest sporting event in the world.

Along with the lack of displayed St. George's flags, you could virtually feel the general sense of people's apathy. It was perfectly justified in all honesty. England had stunk the place out at the previous two tournaments and to put it bluntly, they were a bloody embarrassment to our great nation.

The penny eventually dropped and my decision was made for me during England's first game against Tunisia. A familiar scenario was being played out before me. It was the sight of England 'putting you through the wringer'. It was a circumstance I'd witnessed far too often over the years and it was this rather uncomfortable situation that prompted me to include mine and England's journey in this book.

As a general rule I've always made sure that when watching our national team, it's witnessed along with copious amounts of alcohol. I have found that it helps with the almost guaranteed suffering that you're about to receive when watching England and it does help to soften the blows somewhat. This mission is normally carried out in the safe confines of a crowded pub. This is something else I've also found to help with the pain. We would all turn up in some great misguided sense of optimism, hoping upon hope that England might play well and win. But more often than not, we're left crying into our beer afterwards!

Again, because of my total lack of faith, despite what I've just written, although probably against my better judgement, I decided to watch the match at home from the comfort of my sofa. I knew deep down that I'd probably miss the atmosphere and chaos of the pub. I also knew that I'd miss being soaked in beer if England actually managed to score a goal for some strange reason. However, I was to discover that watching England in a totally sober state is neither sensible nor very good for your health for that matter. It was an experience that I resolved would not be repeated ever again! England managed to win 2-1 despite the best efforts of the referee and in particular, the blind fuckers in the VAR box that were probably stationed at some remote outpost in the deepest darkest depths of Siberia (or perhaps they really should have been considering the lack of help they gave the ref at the time!) I remember thinking after the game that although I'd just made the conscious decision to put pen to paper on the subject of the world cup, our journey in the competition wasn't going to be a long one. The end result would be that I wouldn't have much material to write about anyway!

Away from football, Sian had arranged a lovely surprise for me. She messaged me with a picture that showed a pair of tickets. On these particular tickets, it displayed the name Roddy Radiation and his Skabilly Rebels. Roddy (Roddy Byers) just happens to be a former member of my all-time favourite band The Specials. He was going to be playing in a well-known music venue, The Victoria, in our hometown Swindon. This pub/concert venue always has a very good standard of bands playing there and I along with Sian was really looking forward to the gig. The date for this was to be Saturday 23 June and it was the evening before England's next match against Panama the following day.

Sian and my good self-rocked up at The Victoria just before 7:30 pm for a few 'pre-gig drinks'. We found a table and sat down and just allowed ourselves to take in the atmosphere of this great boozer. We were both very much looking forward to 'a little skank' later, even if my fucked-up knees weren't! As we were sitting there enjoying our drinks some middle-aged gents walked into the pub. If you're of a certain age the sight of what they were wearing was cool and great in equal measure. Fred Perry T-shirts, Ben Sherman shirts, braces holding jeans up, Doc Martens and smart loafers all resulted in a brilliant retro look.

Shortly after, another chap walked in from outside and his attire was a sight to behold. He was wearing a really smart tonic suit, oxblood loafers and good old-fashioned white socks finished off his look, he looked the absolute 'dogs', he really did! We were to find out later that he was actually a member of the support group 'The Erin Bardwell Collective'. For my look, I was fashioned in a 2-tone black and white Ben Sherman short-sleeved shirt, denim shorts (it was summer) summer loafers and of course, finished off with a black leather trilby hat. A lot more old farts like my good self-kept on coming into the pub until eventually before we knew it, it was time for us to make our way to the rear of the building and into the concert room.

As we walked into the fairly large but at the same time intimate feeling room, we saw the support band warming up. Our cool tonic suit attired friend was on the stage checking some equipment. In one corner stood a DJ booth, the guy behind the jump was knocking out all the ska favourites and I could feel my limbs wanting to move already. Standing on the other side of the room was a very well-stocked bar, which was great as it meant you'd miss none of the action. The venue was clean apart from the slightly sticky floor, it had obviously seen a lot of revelry in its time.

As we ordered our drinks the group 'The Erin Bardwell Collective' got going. They played quite a few original ska tracks that had hailed from the very early days of the music genre. They were very good; Sian and I were very impressed.

The group was led by a fantastic female singer and she really could belt out a song, her large booming voice was coming over great. The guy wearing the tonics was playing the keyboards and it wasn't long before lots of young people at heart were dancing, although perhaps their middle-aged limbs were not moving as quickly as they once had!

Along with the ska tracks, the group also played some very upbeat Reggae stuff. Everybody was having a great time and both myself and Sian were 'in the mood'. We were both dancing and I swear that the noise levels were being raised with each passing song. The band did a one-hour set. They were brilliant, but it was time for us old gits to take a break. The drinks flowed too easily once more or perhaps it was all the skanking, we were doing that was making us so thirsty at the time. (That's our excuse anyway!)

With a much-needed pit stopover, it was time for 'Roddy' and his boys to join the party. It's fair to say that we weren't really all that sure what to expect music-wise from the main act. I mean, yeah, okay, there is a clue in the band's title 'The Skabilly Rebels', but ska and rockabilly are a rather unusual combination if indeed that was the type of music that they were potentially going to play. However, we needn't have worried, the Rebels were excellent. They knocked out some The Specials' tracks. These were mainly a mix of some songs that Roddy had actually written for the group and some of the other old favourites. The 'billy side' of their music was a bit hard to explain. I have a brother that is a total rockabilly nut and refuses to listen to anything else, so I'm well acquainted with the 'billy sound'. However, this was certainly different though. The best description I and Sian could come up with at the time was that it seemed a fusion of rockabilly and upbeat country music. Despite our confusion, it needs to be put on record that their particular sound was bloody brilliant. I have since downloaded all of their material at home, I just can't get enough!

Before we had even attended the gig, Sian had given me her usual reliable sage advice concerning my bad knees. As it happens, I'd already decided that I would attempt to go easy on 'the skanking'. Having previously overdone it at the Manchester ska weekend, I wasn't too keen on revisiting that very painful experience. On that occasion, all the skanking had put paid to my shot knees for several weeks afterwards! I did heed Sian's advice, however, and indeed my own and I took it a lot easier, but the problem is that the music just makes you want to jump about, it's just so catchy. (For the record, I did allow myself a couple of full-on skanks.) "See, I can be a good boy sometimes!" Roddy and his Rebel's played with heaps of energy and as I observed around the room that was by now absolutely bouncing, all you could see was a mass of arms and legs moving in all directions, it was fucking mad!

The gig was nearing its end and to be perfectly truthful, so were Sian and I. We were absolutely off our feet, knackered to the point of falling over almost. We made the decision to go and sit in the main bar, we badly needed a well-earned rest. The pub was still very busy, but I found it quite funny that all the people that were sitting in the saloon bar having a nice civilised drink were completely unaware of the madness that was happening further down the corridor. It was two worlds separated by a pair of double doors, quite funny, but strange at the same time. I ordered some more drinks and fortunately for us, a table became available. We both sat there, feeling a bit sore but very contented. It had been a great night, it really had. I'm starting to get a feeling of déjà vu now. A taxi was ordered and we got home and crawled into bed!

Thank you, Sian, for a fantastic night.

NB, I somehow managed to lose my glasses skanking!

It seems there's always a price to pay!

It was Sunday morning, the morning after the night before. I woke up to find that my head was pretty clear and there was no real sign of a much-dreaded hangover, which is always an added bonus. However, my body was telling me I was no longer twenty-one, but it was actually knocking on fifty-three. My decrepit knees were a bit sore, but nonetheless, okay and I had the feeling they were telling me that I really should slow down a tad. (Not like that's ever going to happen!) Sian's aching limbs were also making it known to her that they too were knocking on a bit, but again, on the whole, she was feeling ok.

Our plan for the day was simple, watch the England game and then catch the late afternoon sun in the garden afterwards. The weather on that morning was absolutely gorgeous once again, what a brilliant summer we'd been blessed with. The sunbathing after the match was only ever going to go two ways in my mind 1. I would be sat in my chair in the garden with a big grin on my face because England had just won and at the same time holding a large glass of gin and tonic (I know, I've joined the gin club too!) or two. Sat in the same said chair with a long face and trying to pull what little is left of my hair out in utter frustration at what was another crap England performance. (And possibly with an even larger glass of gin and tonic in hand to drown my sorrows.)

My prematch concerns, however, turned out to be completely unwarranted on that glorious Sunday afternoon. What transpired took me and no doubt the rest of the watching population by complete surprise. England thrashed a very poor Panama side 6-1! I say poor, but poor is perhaps a slight understatement when describing that South American side. I'm personally of the opinion that they'd be lucky to survive in the championship in our domestic league, but having said that, nothing should be taken away from England's performance. In the first half, their play and finishing were very clinical and it was a joy to watch. I'm also sure if that they hadn't taken their foot off the gas, a score of double figures may well have been reached, but maybe I'm being a little bit unkind towards our opponents as they did up their game slightly in the second half. Regardless of all of this, that result certainly wasn't in the script and not a score line you'd expect to see at the world cup finals. Suffice to say, the sunbathing and copious amounts of gin drunk afterwards were fervently enjoyed very much by the two of us.

Move Along, Please. There's Nothing to See Here!

The statement above best describes England's third and final group game against Belgium. It was basically a dead rubber as both sides had already qualified for the knockout stages. The only thing riding on the game was who would win the group and who would end up second. This had a final bearing as to which half of the draw the two nations were placed. The match itself was a total bore-fest and was played out with all the intensity of a testimonial game and it bored me rigid! One piece of brilliance finally settled the match in

Belgium's favour and it was they who won the group and were placed in the supposed tougher half of the draw.

A much-changed England side seemed to lack the desire for a positive result and you did wonder if they even wanted to be out on the pitch at all! The England manager had stated to the media that England would go all out for the win and finish top of the group, but to anybody who had the misfortune to watch the game would have to disagree, however. Perhaps mind-poker games were being played out, I can't say for sure, but it was all irrelevant in the grand scheme of things as far as I was concerned because now the knock-out stages were beginning and we would now witness 'real games' that really would have something important resting on the outcome.

Columbia Awaits!

I am sometimes accused of being too cynical, but the second-round match against Columbia turned out exactly how I'd envisaged beforehand. The previous game against Belgium had been a 'borefest' whereas the coming together against the South Americans ultimately turned into a 'kick fest'! South American teams will very often employ dirty underhand tactics to win games. This match was no exception and our cause wasn't helped because a very weak and out of his depth American referee had been appointed to officiate proceedings. This match always had the potential to turn into an explosive powder keg and with only a few minutes into the game having passed, my worst fears were confirmed. England were trying to play football but were being continually frustrated by the Columbian's cynical tackling and I was getting more and more wound up by what was happening out on the pitch. My bad mood was to reach fever point just before half time. I can only think that headbutting an opponent must be an accepted part of the game where this lot were from because as the defensive wall was being lined, a Columbian player literally headbutted one of our players. "What the fuck?" I screamed, "That's a red card ref!" Now, the whole world and his wife couldn't have failed to spot that offence, it was so blatant and a downright disgusting act that had no belonging whatsoever on a football pitch.

I was to end up lost for words, however. It seemed that we had the misfortune to have the very same blind fuckers sat in the VAR box as we'd had in the Tunisia match. Not one of them had spotted the incident, it was unbelievable, how the hell could they have not seen that! I felt cheated and very angry at the injustice of it all. The feeling I had in the pit of my stomach was all too familiar to me and I just wanted it to go away. You couldn't even blame our American cousin on that occasion for not spotting the headbutt as he had his hands full at the time trying to stop all of the other shenanigans that were being employed by the dirty Columbians.

The dirty cynical fouls, descent and just general confrontation towards the ref, unfortunately, continued into the second half until at long last some overdue justice towards England was served. We were awarded a penalty, however, this failed to stop the Columbian's dirty tricks. They wouldn't clear the penalty area and they just continued to remonstrate with the ref over his decision. But worst of all, as all this commotion was going on, a Columbian player was deliberately scuffing up the penalty spot! (What were those extra officials doing in the VAR box at the time?) You really do have to wonder!

A full three minutes, 'yes, three minutes!' had elapsed before captain Harry was allowed to confidently dispatch the penalty home. He really did show nerves of steel in the face of all that provocation and gamesmanship to score that all-important goal. Our very young side were having to grow up fast, many of them had probably never played in a game of that nature, but they were holding out against all the South Americans could throw at them. I felt very proud of them, but at the same time, I was finding myself getting more angry. That South American team were literally stinking the world cup out and more to the point, they were dragging the beautiful game down into the gutter. I really felt at the time that our brave young lads were going to hold out for the win, but the footballing gods had other ideas. A last-minute, totally undeserved equaliser by the Columbians ensured that extra time beckoned. "Fuck, fuck, fuck!" For the second time that evening, I'd been left speechless, I couldn't believe it. *How could the footballing gods allow such injustice*, I thought.

I really don't like extra time, I never have. More often than not very little action occurs as most teams seem to adopt the mindset that the game is going to end in penalties anyway. Of course, deep down I was praying that hope upon hope that England would nick a goal and save me from the mental torture of the dreaded penalty shoot-out. I have over the years had the terrible misfortune of witnessing England lose six penalty shoot-outs. The one and only successful time I've seen the three lions prevail was against Spain at Euro '96, so as you can imagine.

I was very keen on a positive result in the 120 minutes of play. My prayers weren't answered, however, no further goals scored meant only one outcome and an outcome that I wanted no part of whatsoever! I made a promise to myself after the last time England lost on penalties that I'd never again put myself through all that torture and heartbreak. I turned the TV off and took myself off to bed. Some younger fans might well recoil in horror at my actions, I'd probably be of the same opinion not that many years ago, but for the sake of my sanity and general wellbeing, I now respectively decline any invitation to watch an England penalty shoot-out.

As I laid on the top of my bed, I did temporarily think that I must be barking, but that thought didn't last long. As it turned out I could hear all that was happening anyway. We live within spitting distance of our old local pub and because it was a warm night all the windows were open. Sian's not a fan of penalties either, so she was lying next to me. We couldn't really tell exactly what was going on. We were hearing cheers and groans, but were they cheers for an England goal or a save by our keeper?

This agonising situation carried on for some time and to be honest, I was finding it only slightly less stressful than I had been watching it myself. However, all of a sudden, a cheer rang out that was so much louder than all that'd come before. "Bloody hell! England must have won," I shouted out to Sian. She then raced downstairs to check the TV.

"Yeah, they've won, Phil," came Sian's booming voice via the stairs. It was an unbelievable feeling to finally win a world cup game in those circumstances. It did feel good, but also strange in a way and for a few moments, I did wish that we'd been out somewhere watching it all unfold and getting soaked in beer, it would've been brilliant.

After getting so hyped up over the game, it took me ages to get off to sleep. However, it gave me the chance to think about my decision to physically not watch all of the drama. I felt totally vindicated and I had no doubts that I'd done the right thing and I will do the same again if the situation arises. (Although no more penalty shoot-outs please!)

Bring on Sweden!

The summer of 1976, oops, I meant to say 2018 was still blissfully continuing on its merry way as I awoke on that very sunny and warm Saturday morning. Obviously, one of the very first thoughts that'd entered my head as I attempted to drag my old bones out of bed concerned the little matter of England's quarterfinal match against Sweden later that afternoon. Under normal circumstances, I would've felt quite nervous about a game of that magnitude, but for some reason, I felt we were going to get past Sweden without too much drama. I took the very short walk across the road to my local convenience store. I needed some supplies of beer for the match and I picked up my daily copy of the current bun (*The Sun*). The headlines on the back page concerning England's chances of winning the game were, I felt, still of a slightly restrained nature. It's fair to say that most of the general sporting public are more than well aware just how the tabloids used to whip unmerited public hysteria when it comes to our national football team, but that just hadn't been the case at this tournament.

In fact, the expectations from our 'red tops' were realistically much lower than they'd ever been and were perhaps rightly so. England's performances in the last two or three tournaments had been so woeful that it had caused everybody's hopes to crash and burn in no uncertain terms. To further prove my point, before the competition had even started *The Sun* had printed a cartoon depicting the England team's aeroplane parked up in a short-stay car park, it was fucking hilarious! And an accurate measure of the nation's expectations at Russia 2018.

Thankfully, the hours leading up to the game pass by rather quickly and before you knew it, it was three o'clock and time for the kick-off. As I've already said, I felt we were going to win the game, but I also knew that it wasn't going to be a walk in the park. Previous matches against Sweden had always proved difficult and what they may lack in skill is often replaced with team organisation and lots of effort. The game certainly didn't have the same drama as the kick fest against Columbia had proved and the first twenty-five/thirty minutes had turned out to be a rather uneventful affair, i.e. until England won a corner. A perfect cross is met by 'slab head', who rises above everybody else to power home a perfect header, "Yes, get in there!" 1-0. England added another in the 58th minute and we were cruising. Sweden to be fair had to come into the game at some point and we had to be very thankful to our young goalkeeper from Washington Tyne and Wear for keeping the Swedes at bay. He pulled off three stunning saves in that second half to keep the score line at 2-0 and England made it through to the world cup semi-final.

With the summer sun still blazing away outside, Sian and I retreated to the garden. We both soaked up the late afternoon sunshine. But if truth be told, I was soaking up England's 2-0 win and it felt great. We were in our first world cup semi-final for twenty-eight years. It had been a very long wait with lots of heartache in between, so I for one couldn't wait for the game to come. For some strange reason all of my beer supplies had bitten the dust, so my gin club membership card was stamped once again! Talking about gin, we were on that occasion drinking from a bottle that had been a present from one of Sian's friends. They had been away on holiday and had very kindly brought us this very nice gin. It was called Tanqueray and was export strength and it blew your socks off!

Suffice to say that Saturday evening was spent in a somewhat blurry state and neither Sian nor I can recall many details. (Oh well, such is life!) We were going to have to sweat it out for four days, four days that gave me far too much time to consider all the possible outcomes. Unlike the Sweden game where I'd felt confident of a successful result, I can only say that before the semi-final against Croatia, I wasn't quite carrying the same level of faith as before for some reason.

Croatia Awaits!

We Get the Bullet! Part 2

It's exactly one week since we bit the bullet and tumbled out of the 2018 Russian world cup. To be perfectly honest with you, it's taken me a whole week to summon up the will to put pen to paper again. I've now had the misfortune to witness England losing a major semi-final for the third time and it hurts, it really hurts! To further compound my troubles I suffered a setback concerning my mental wellbeing which threw me off course during that week. I will go more into detail regarding that situation in the next chapter. The most upsetting aspect of England's defeat to Croatia for me was the fact that once again, they'd managed to rescue defeat from the jaws of victory. World champions of throwing games away perhaps? On this occasion, I feel no urgent need to retell any of the details of the match. A game of that magnitude would almost certainly have been watched by anybody interested in the proceedings, even if they were not the biggest of football fans normally. Because of the agony of yet another semi-final defeat, I was doing everything I could to erase the painful memories of that night, but it was proving nigh on impossible. It just kept on haunting my thoughts and it wouldn't leave me alone no matter how hard I tried.

Credit must be given to England's manager though. He has taken us forward after so many years of doom and gloom and I feel that this is just the start of great success to come (fingers crossed!) I always used to tell myself that the next tournament would be ours and that it would be our turn for the glory, but so far, it's failed to materialise. Four years is a heck of a long time to wait for things to go right on the pitch and I've had the above thought for forty plus years now! I often wonder if I'll ever see an England captain lift that wonderful gold trophy aloft above their head ever again! Many years ago, I recall a conversation over a beer with my brother, Rich (the brother I'd stayed with during my separation with Sian). We both agreed on that occasion that we'd both die very happy men if we could witness England winning the world cup just one more time. However, he then reminded me that I had been lucky enough to see this happen the first time around. "Oh yeah, but I was only nine months old at the time!" I replied. Cheeky git!

France went on to win the competition and deservedly so. As much as it pains me to say, they were the best team at the tournament and richly merited their status as the best team in the world. I think it's fair to say that there had been quite a bit of apprehension before the start of the 2018 Russian world cup. Worries of major trouble involving Russian football hooligans, thankfully, never surfaced and the whole showpiece was a resounding success. It was brilliantly organised with wonderful stadiums and all the attending nations played in a manner that told you that they seemed very intent on making this competition a great sporting spectacle (all except Columbia!). The Russian citizens can feel very proud of the way they hosted that great sporting event. It did make me wonder if other people's ingrained perceptions in regard to the Russian population might have changed. I know that my own thoughts and opinions had altered. My earlier preconceptions towards the country of the big brown bear had definitely been blown out of the water forever.

The one and only thought that I was able to take comfort from after England's semi-final defeat was the fact that at least on this occasion, they hadn't stunk the tournament out as they had done in recent history. Those very young lads returned as heroes and the future for our national team does indeed look bright. England are world cup holders at U-17 and U-20 age group level and are European champions at another. So, who knows maybe, just maybe, this old fart will get to see his wish come true. Time will always tell!

Chapter Twenty-Five
My Black Dog Turns Vicious!

I made a brief reference in regards to my mental health wellbeing in the previous chapter. My reaction to England's semi-final loss was bad, really bad in fact. The anger and frustration I felt were totally off the scale and I'd turned into someone I certainly didn't recognise and more to the point, I didn't like whatsoever! I was literally screaming all sorts of offensive obscenities in the direction of the poor old TV screen. It wasn't its fault obviously, but I had to vent my pent-up frustration at something and I certainly didn't want it to be the love of my whole life, Sian. Sian decided to take herself off to bed as she was absolutely disgusted with my behaviour and I for one didn't blame her one little bit. I was being vile and repulsive and I wouldn't have wanted to be around me at that time either.

Some small sensible part of my brain suggested to me that it would be a good idea to get out of that situation and so I decided to take myself off and go and sit in the garden. I was to find that yet again, it was another lovely summer evening as I sat down in the recliner chair. I sat there for what seemed like hours just gawping up to the sky, a sky that was slowly turning into the night with the stars beginning to shine through. Some of these stars were already twinkling and the whole sky looked beautiful, although to me at that time, this incredible sight looked anything but wondrous! The incidents of the match kept on going over and over again in my head. It was proving impossible to shut it out. The what ifs, if only they'd done that etc. we're bouncing from one side of my head to the other. It was driving me fucking nuts, it really was!

All of this was making me really angry and pissed off. I kept on asking some mysterious person or force from up above in the heavens, "Why does it always end like this, just for once, can't it go our way?" Looking back now, the idea that somebody was ever going to answer me seems rather ridiculous. I certainly don't believe in God and I'm not religious in any shape or form, so whom I was trying to talk to is a complete mystery to me.

I mentioned previously (session 16) that I was becoming somewhat impatient regarding my perceived recovery. I've given the matter a lot of thought. I was very concerned at the way I'd reacted to England's loss. Previous disappointments had left me feeling a bit flat and generally pissed off for a few days, but my actions on that occasion were completely over the top and outside the boundaries of my normal behaviour. I came to the conclusion that these events had coincided with what I now know as 'one of my small bumps in the road'.

At the beginning of July 18, I'd started getting symptoms, anger symptoms. These were by no means big but they were making me aware of their existence. I wasn't overly concerned by this, however, I had after all experienced these small blips before during the journey on the road of my recovery and I was pretty convinced that this was just another hurdle I had to negotiate. I now suspect that my 'perceived impatience' and the start of my 'anger issues' were linked and unfortunately for me, the timing of England's defeat compounded this particular 'small bump' to a level which I wasn't ready for or more to the point, effectively armed emotionally to constructively deal with.

A bolt from the blue is the only way to best describe the emotional fallout I experienced after England's semi-final defeat. It shook my already fragile foundations and I really did feel disgusted at my over the top negative actions. This alone was bad enough, but what was concerning me more was that it felt as though all of my good work regarding my recovery had all been undone by this one event. I was really pissed off. I'd been working so hard to get well again and it felt as though I'd let myself down big time. It's worth noting that I had expressed to Isobel during a very recent session that I had this nagging thought in the back of my mind that 'things' regarding my recovery were in fact, I thought, 'going too well'. It certainly felt at the time that my house of cards had come crashing down around my ears and that I was back at square one. The thought of starting all over again absolutely terrified me. I didn't feel I had the will or indeed the energy to start the fight with that demonic depression monster once again.

Obviously, I didn't want to be proved right on this. I knew deep down inside of me that I was probably catastrophising the whole issue, but what was to follow in the next four or five days did little to convince me otherwise! My anger monster had woken from his slumber and he was positively raging with anger. The intensity of my anger was on a level that I probably hadn't felt since my very early teens. It was at this time, if you remember, that I'd suffered bullying at senior school. This had happened very close timewise to the sexual abuse I received from my father. I did wonder if all this anger was tied in. I was well aware that after my counselling sessions I'd experienced 'small blips' regarding the relevant issues that had been raised between Isobel and me. These small emotional hiccups had always been dealt with in a very good positive manner and any physical or mental symptoms would normally dissipate themselves within a few days. But any aftershocks concerning anger had never manifested themselves.

My anger issues had been covered in great detail during counselling and I would wait with bated breath afterwards for some kind of reaction, but it just never happened! This was making me very worried indeed. I had effectively opened up a very serious mental can of worms and I'd been walking around for some time with a large gaping wound that was bleeding profusely. All of my pent-up anger and frustration concerning the abuse and bullying that desperately needed to escape my soul was, for some unseen reason, not being permitted to happen. However, the ticking time bomb finally exploded after England's defeat. Looking back now, I happen to think that it could have been any painful situation that would have ultimately tipped me over the edge and into the abyss. As much as I love football, I know that it's not a matter of life or death and as I've previously stated, normally, I'd be just a bit flat for a few days that's all and certainly not be the very angry vile person that surfaced at that horrible time.

For the record, I have to state that none of my anger was taken out on Sian. I gave her the silent treatment, just like I always had. This is an issue that's always been a bone of contention between us. Sian wants me to talk to her when I'm feeling rough and when I'm okay, I say, "Yes, next time I'll talk to you." The thing is that I really wish I could find the energy to speak to her when I'm bad because it does make me feel like complete shit.

The problem is my demon is so bloody strong that I've only ever got enough will and vigour to fight him and nothing else! On this occasion especially, I was just so desperate to tell her how I felt that 1. The total shock at my behaviour. 2. Sad that I felt I was back to square one. 3. So, so angry that my head was all over the place. 4. Felt disheartened that I'd given into my demon. 5. Was giving 110% to all of the elements that were needed to realise my recovery, but someone or something was doing its level best to keep me down.

As I've previously clarified, the levels of anger within me at that time were so bad they were actually scaring the living daylights out of me. The four or five very angry days that followed our exit from the Russian world cup were utterly awful in the extreme. Mr Very, Very Angry would be the best way to describe my mood and demeanour during those pain-filled days. It really didn't matter what I was doing either. Simple tasks such as making a brew, washing up and hoovering were proving impossible to undertake without using foul language all of the time. I would be shouting and screaming at the top of my voice at the poor kettle, telling it to hurry the fuck up. I just wanted my cup of rosy and I wanted it now! (How fucked up is that!) Nothing was allowed to escape from my vile outbursts, crazy I know, but that's how bad I was suffering at that time. It really did feel as if I was fighting an ongoing daily battle with some very nasty entity that I was unable to see. In hindsight, it was logical to assume that it was most probably my old demon foe that was stirring up all of my hatred and anger. He was the only one capable of inflicting all that venom on to me, he's such an evil vicious bastard!

Due to the excellent summer, we were having, I was able to spend a lot of time sitting in the garden during those pain-racked days. I continued to sit and just stare up into the heavens, hoping for some possible enlightenment, but of course, I never did receive an answer to any of my questions. (Funny that!) All of the constant mental infighting that I was enduring was beginning to take its toll on me. I was getting tired and it was all I could do to just keep a lid on my anger when Sian returned home from work. The one and only thought that I kept having while all of this shit was going on was the possibility that finally, at last, my bottled up hurt and anger was being allowed to pour out of my very damaged soul. I had waited so long for that to happen if this was the case. I gleaned some comfort from the fact that what I'd been through would at least have been worth all the pain and suffering I'd endured if it meant that I was finally ridding myself of my greatest foe.

When I started the counselling process back in January 2018, I was more than well aware that I was going to be stirring up the proverbial hornet's nest. I really had no idea what kind of experience would greet me. (Who would?) At times it's often felt as if I'm nervously stepping through an emotional minefield, while at the same time trying to pick the right spots whilst wearing a blindfold! Adding to all of this has been the constant hits or what I very fondly describe as my 'small bumps in the road'. I remember telling Isobel during a previous session that at times it was almost as if I was back at school. The counselling process with all the many different issues that had been raised, which had, in turn, caused me to experience a lot of emotional fallout, had actually made me seriously question everything again. Instead of learning subjects like maths and English, you wake up each day thinking what am I going to learn about myself today?

Thankfully, my utterly vile anger symptoms did slowly dissipate and in the end, my illness showed me some grace and long overdue compassion. It had taken roughly a week for me to feel any semblance of calm again. The anger had been merciless and unforgiving. It had tried its very best to floor me, but I was still standing (just) and it really did feel like I'd come through something terrible and that I was now looking at it from the other side.

Chapter Twenty-Six
Session 17, Signing Off

My next visit to Bradford House took place after an enforced three-week break due to Isobel's holiday. Unfortunately, I hadn't been able to take full advantage of this short holiday, this was because during that time, I was experiencing some small anger aftershocks. These 'hits' had a small negative impact on me, but thankfully, no long-lasting damage was meted out on my still somewhat fragile disposition.

Isobel greeted me and once again welcomed me inside that wonderful Victorian property. As I sat down in the chair in that rather plain non-descript room, I realised that in fact, I'd not missed it one little bit. If anything, all it seemed to do was to remind me of all pain and suffering that had occurred during my past sessions with Isobel. "Hello, Phil, how have you been?" I paused for a bit, I was a bit reluctant to answer her, to be honest.

In the week leading up to this appointment, I'd been slightly worried about facing up to Isobel because of what I saw as my perceived setback in my recovery. I knew that this idea I had in my head was totally stupid and I couldn't understand exactly why I felt that way. After all, it wasn't as if Isobel was going to tell me off like some naughty schoolboy who hadn't done his homework. If anything, her reaction to me would be the same as it always was' warm, reassuring and totally non-judgemental.

I poured out to Isobel all of the grisly details concerning the anger issues that had plagued me since our last appointment together. "The anger dam had finally ruptured and I was utterly powerless to stop it." I went further, "It just had to come out, all the brown bile that spewed out was affectively all of my bottled up fury and frustration and the many decades of sheer, sheer anger that I was made to live with was literally gushing out of my battle-scarred soul".

I could sense in Isobel's demeanour that she knew I'd been struggling with all of this. She was, as always, kind and compassionate in her response and she offered up a comforting but very pertinent fact to me. "You've come so far in such a relatively short space of time, Phil. You should be congratulating yourself. You really have progressed well in your recovery and the anger blips are part and parcel of the whole process." My lovely counsellor was spot on and of course, I was only too well aware of this fact, but sometimes everybody needs some words of encouragement thrown in their way and at that time, I certainly needed a figurative arm around my shoulder.

I had long suspected that the emotional fallout from my anger problems was always very likely to inflict on me the worst possible of reactions. Having said that, however, the cataclysmic levels of my angst and fury took me by complete surprise and it really left me in an appalling state of shock. I really had long forgotten all about the vicious temper that I used to possess and the thought of it returning frightened the life out of me. The bad temper was never likely to be played out on anybody; I must stress. But that person that was me at that horrible time was somebody I didn't recognise, didn't recognise at all. I say this because these days, I consider myself to be a mild-mannered middle-aged bloke that no longer goes looking for trouble, but the reflection I saw of myself in the mirror what not something very pleasing on the eye, in fact, the image absolutely repulsed me.

Isobel enquired as to whether I thought my anger had passed. "No, I don't, not entirely, it's definitely subsiding, but it's still there to some degree, things that don't normally bother me do and that's how I know it's not left me completely," I replied. I added to this by saying, "I'm always very wary. If there is one sure thing, I can be certain of, it is that little demon fucker is lurking somewhere in some dark corner of my mind, waiting to ambush me when I least suspect it."

Isobel gave me a rather quizzical look, "what do you mean exactly when you say that?"

"He will sit back and wait in the background, almost as if he is stalking me and when he sees me getting happy and well again and making good progress in my life, the sick fuck will strike again, hitting me with everything in his Armor. In the past he would totally floor me, but not anymore!" I took a deep breath and then I took an even bigger sip of water from my glass. It was a very hot day and my mouth was as dry as Gandhi's thongs, the Sahara Desert and a nun's habit all rolled into one.

I went on to explain that my demon is no longer able to deliver the knockout blow. He tries, but he now meets his match. As I've got better, the natural strength inside of me has increased to the extent that I've now got the ability to skilfully fend him off. Having said all of that, however, I felt I needed to explain to Isobel that I obviously wasn't completely out of the woods just yet. There was still a fight going on. On one of my shoulders, I had a guardian angel, he'd forever be telling me that I was strong, in fact, I was stronger than I'd ever realised. He would constantly reassure me, telling me to not get discouraged at times, I was doing everything in my power to get well again. He'd scream at the top of his voice at me, "Just give yourself a break, Phil!" The devil on my other shoulder would dismiss all of this with his usual disdain, but with every passing day, his voice becomes weaker, no longer loud and inflammatory, but more like a pitiful heart-rending echo coming from a nearly defeated foe.

A few awkward moments of silence followed until Isobel asked, "Are you okay, Phil?"

"Yeah, yeah, I'm okay, just a bit mentally tired that's all, I'm fine." It was nearing the end of the session once again. We both decided it would be unwise to call a halt to the counselling at that time. The plan was to carry on for at least another six weeks, I considered them to be 'maintenance sessions'. All of the heavy groundwork had been covered, but there had been and probably still were 'small bumps in the road to negotiate'.

This chapter is called *'Signing Off'* as it will be the last session entry in this book. It was without question the hardest task that I've ever undertaken in my whole life. I apologise if the subject matter regarding my sessions with the lovely Isobel has made for heavy reading, but it was a necessary part of my journey and a very important aspect of my story that I felt needed to be told. As I've already stated before, this book was written in the prime hope that it can maybe be of help to other people that are suffering from mental health problems. If there is one significant point that they can identify and take away with them and can help them on their road to recovery, then all of the effort it took me to write this publication will have been worth all of the many hours I've put in to make it happen.

Epilogue

Come on, hands up, who of you out there have ever found yourself singing along to one of your favourite tracks thinking that the words you're singing back are the correct ones and for whatever reason later, you find out that maybe one or two words of the lyrics are completely different to what you imagine are being sung? I ask this question because just recently I became an honourable member of 'the misheard song lyric club'. For thirty plus years, I was utterly convinced the above-mentioned words in the title of this chapter that were part of a track made famous by '80s pop group Aztec Camera called *'Somewhere in My Heart'* were, to all intents and purposes, the exact words I thought I always heard whenever the song was played on the radio.

Sian, after looking up for research purposes discovered that what was actually being sung on that hit record was 'an ambition of love' and not 'a vision of love'. I have to state for the record that when she'd informed me of that not so little fact, my chin went on to hit the floor in no uncertain terms. I just couldn't believe it; I felt such a fool. Sian told me not to worry as she thought 'my version' made for a good chapter title heading anyway. All of this is rather odd in a bizarre way. From the very first occasion that I ever heard the song, those standout words had, excuse the pun, struck a chord with me. I've absolutely no idea why this happened, for some strange reason it just did! To further emphasise my point, I neither like nor dislike the song or the group for that matter, they just weren't my thing. However, I've always loved that line from that track and it has managed to stay with me to this very day.

I tell myself that for some crazy reason, the words were going to be important to me and that one day they were going to serve a very significant purpose. When I took the decision to start writing this book, I was always happy with the knowledge that I had in fact, the perfect title for my final chapter. The fact I'm writing at all is thanks in part to Mel. It had been her suggestion in the first place that I should put pen to paper and tell my story. Some twelve months before meeting Mel, I really couldn't have contemplated taking on a project such as this. So once again, I thank you, Mel, for giving me the belief and confidence that I could actually sit down and attempt to write my first book.

The words I've highlighted that pertain to the song, *'Somewhere in My Heart',* I feel fully describes and encapsulates the magical adventure, the whole odyssey of myself and Sian's very happy and joyful but often troubled time together. In a metaphorical sense, the boxing gloves represent my 'little friend', the demon. He has consistently jabbed away at my very being, causing me to suffer no end of pain. He inflicted many severe knockout blows on my very fragile soul. And this, in turn, would make me endure so many numerous days of depressive concussion. His punches got even more powerful around the time that Sian and I first started our relationship. There was no blame attached to Sian, no culpability was transmitted from her direction whatsoever.

It was just the simple fact that my own personal circumstances had obviously changed dramatically. And the fallout because of all this turned out to be horrendous. The most upsetting issue I had trouble dealing with at that time was the very sudden change in the state of affairs regarding my relationship with my son and daughter. As you're now well aware, the situation with my ex-wife became very bitter and volatile after out separation, which eventually resulted in me having a total non-existent relationship with my kids.

That damaging and very upsetting situation I found myself in had such a negative impact on me, but more to the point, it was causing catastrophic injury to Sian and the extremely early bloom of our relationship. I am now 100% certain in my mind that the issues surrounding myself and my children and the subsequent consequences that followed were the catalyst for the onset of my very serious depression problems. Those rather symbolic boxing gloves have caused so much unspeakable destruction. They have so much to answer for, they really do!

'*Singing Hearts and Flowers*' fully describes and encompasses the opposite end of our relationship spectrum. In between the dark periods, there have been many very happy times. Some of which I've chronicled in this publication. At various times my depression has tended to overshadow these happy events, such is the nature of my illness. You have to realise and take into account that even when there are periods when I've been very well, the depressive poison that is forever infecting my system never totally goes away. As I've got well, I've been able to better manage my condition. The stronger I've got, the easier it has become, but I have to acknowledge the stark fact that this illness I've been blessed with will, unfortunately for me, be an affliction, I will perhaps always have to live with.

Having said that, however, I repeat, Sian and I have had some really great times together. We've enjoyed holidays abroad, lots of short breaks and many, many booze-filled episodes. (Although this has subsided somewhat due to our age!) *'Singing Hearts and Flowers'* also represents to me our love, affection, friendship and ultimately our lifetime of love that we've always had for one another. Sian has always had a small piece of my heart and for whatever reason, I knew that she was going to play a major part in my life again. Our coming together again after so many years apart is a true modern-day fairy tale and solid proof that love really can conquer all.

My old adversary, the demon, has tried everything within his power to destroy all that Sian and I have built up over the years. He has been utterly relentless in his quest to annihilate the pair of us. But we have stood toe to toe with him, taken everything his wickedness has thrown at us, felt all the painful blows both mentally and physically, sailed through vicious storms that have threatened to shipwreck us, but yet, here we are, still able to stand upright with our constitutions uncommonly strong.

I will for the foreseeable future carry on participating in my sessions with Isobel. The autumn months are just around the corner and historically speaking, it can be quite hard for me. It will be interesting to see how I react and cope with these sometimes rather gloomy months. However, I can confidently state that I do now feel much stronger and better equipped to deal with any potential thumps and bumps that may well appear from over the distant horizon. What life has in store for me in my immediate future is slightly unclear and I couldn't begin to speculate.

I'm still taking one day at a time, it's all I can do and to be perfectly fair. This approach up till now has served me very well. I continue to improve and get stronger with each passing day, but you've come to realise by now that I'm still very cautious, I have to be. I have to be vigilant and stay on my toes as you never know if and when my old enemy will attempt to strike next. I can't pretend that it's anything but fucking hard work and it can be incredibly frustrating at times. But there is one fact I can categorically state. I am winning the war and perhaps one day I will get to live a depression free life. Sian and I will raise a glass, or two, to that!